Community-Based Systems of Long Term Care

Community-Based Systems of Long Term Care

Rick T. Zawadski, PhD
Editor

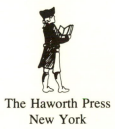

The Haworth Press
New York

Community-Based Systems of Long Term Care has also been published as *Home Health Care Services Quarterly,* Volume 4, Numbers 3/4, Fall/Winter 1983.

The Haworth Press, Inc., 28 East 22 Street, New York, NY 10010

Library of Congress Cataloging in Publication Data
Main entry under title:

Community-based systems of long term care.

"Home health care services quarterly, volume 4, numbers 3/4."
Includes bibliographies.
1. Long-term care of the sick—United States. 2. Community health services—United States. 3. Community health services for the aged—United States. I. Zawadski, Rick T. II. Home health care services quarterly.
RA644.6.C66   1984   362.1'6   83-22703
ISBN 0-86656-255-9

Community-Based Systems of Long Term Care

Home Health Care Services Quarterly
Volume 4, Numbers 3/4

CONTENTS

PART III
BRINGING IT TOGETHER—A BEGINNING

JANET E. STARR, BS. *Executive Director, Home Care Association of New York State, Inc., Syracuse, New York*

MONNICA C. STEWART, MB, BS, D(Obst), RCOG, *Community Medicine Physician, City and East London Area Health Authority, London, United Kingdom*

ANN-MARIE THOM, *Executive Director, Visiting Nurse Association of New York, New York*

PATRICIA THOMAS, *Executive Director, Visiting Homemakers Association, Toronto, Ontario, Canada*

JUDITH LA VOR WILLIAMS, *Florence Heller School for Advanced Studies in Social Welfare, Brandeis University, Waltham, Massachusetts*

Acknowledgements

While my name is the only one that appears as editor on the cover of this book, the work within reflects the contributions of many people. I would like to first acknowledge and thank a person who rightfully should be designated co-editor, Carol Van Steenberg. Carol assisted and advised in every phase of this work. Her mark, in many cases a good deal of her work, has gone into every page of every chapter, but most of all I appreciate Carol's support and encouragement in what at times has been a very difficult task.

I'd like to, in addition, thank the support staff at On Lok, in particular Sue Wong and Chris van Reenen. These two people entered almost every word in the word processing system and made all of the changes that inevitably were required. Their late hours and weekend work was above the call of duty and I hope this work is deserving of their dedication and their efforts. Jackie Waldman also deserves special mention for keeping track of all the tables and figures and providing her insights through review and editing.

I would also like to thank the authors who participated in this volume. Most of the authors are service providers—involved with the development and operation of a demonstration program—who took time away from their programs to describe their projects and experiences. Each of these authors was asked to follow a very defined outline, to address very many detailed issues, to focus and develop a theme issue and to do all of this within a very tight timeframe. I thank the authors for their participation and their cooperation in this effort. I think that the readers will agree that these authors collectively provide many years of experience in community based-services and that their chapters reflect an understanding of the practical and policy issues in long term care. I only hope that the integrating chapters preceding and following the project chapters do justice to their contributions.

Special thanks are also due to Laura Reif and Brahna Trager, the editors of the *Home Health Care Services Quarterly* for their support of this effort. Not only did they provide an opportunity for this monograph by making available the space in their journal, but they provided advice and encouragement throughout the writing and went out of their way to facilitate the production of the volume in a timely fashion. One thing that did become clear in assembling this volume was these editors' understanding that home health care is a broad topic area encompassing all community-based programs of long term care; they have demonstrated that their journal is the proper forum for this important new field.

Last but not least, I'd like to thank my wife Margaret and my children, Elizabeth and Michael, for the many lost weekends and abbreviated vacations and their patience, without which, this book would not have come into being.

Rick T. Zawadski

Preface

Addressing a major topic like "community-based systems of long term care" is a humbling experience. First, there are literally hundreds of long term care demonstrations in this country, but only a few could be featured. Second, in an area where innovation is the watchword, the target is ever-moving. Even as drafts were being prepared for this work, scores of changes were occurring—in state and federal legislation, in available research data, in the projects themselves.

Consequently, this effort is designed to communicate sharply and clearly—as a snapshot—a particular view of community-based long term care in the early 1980s. It is not so much meant to provide the last word in community care as to give the reader a new way to look at the developments of the last decades and access current movements in this arena.

It should also be noted that this volume is not intended to be an account prepared by disinterested third parties—the perspective is a view from inside. That is, the chroniclers all are persons who developed innovative demonstration programs and then administered them. As guest editor for this volume I decided that such a "first person" record was long overdue even if it meant giving up some objectivity in order to capture our realities.

As you read through this volume you will learn about a variety of approaches and about our convictions related to community-based long term care—mine, as editor, will come through most strongly and consistently. To my colleagues who have contributed their stories but who do not necessarily share all my views, I offer my gratitude for their patience and tolerance.

Rick T. Zawadski

Community-Based Systems of Long Term Care

PART I

BACKGROUND OF LONG TERM CARE

Introduction

In the 1970s, a revolution in services to the aged took place. Consumers—the aged and their families—and service providers screamed out for more effective systems to meet the service needs of the growing population of frail aged. In response to these cries, demonstration projects were begun across the country. While different in their design and methods of operation, all these demonstrations sought to integrate services to reflect more closely the needs of their populations. In addition, these demonstrations tended to emphasize the use of community-based services instead of institutional services, and in most cases, the programs had a primary objective—the control of long term health care costs. Now, with many of these demonstrations having completed at least one and in some cases two or more stages of evolution, it is time to step back and learn from these programs the answers as well as some of the new questions relating to the development of comprehensive coordinated community-based systems of long term care.

In Part II, the planners and charismatic leaders who developed these demonstration projects describe their programs and some of the lessons they learned. In Part III, a theoretical framework is presented for use in the systematic comparison of the projects; the projects' research findings are interpreted; and the policy implications of these demonstrations are discussed. But to set the stage for these presentations, Part I describes the milieu from which these projects sprung.

Chapter 1

The Long Term Care Demonstration Projects: What Are They and Why They Came into Being

Rick T. Zawadski, PhD

In the first part of this chapter, we look at some of the problems of traditional long term care which motivated the development of the community-based demonstration projects addressed by this monograph. Next the development of some alternative services within long term care and the evolution of long term care systems are described. The last part of the chapter focuses directly on the systems interventions represented by the projects included in this monograph and outlines three basic models that can be distinguished among the demonstrations.

WHY ALTERNATIVES?—THE PROBLEM WITH TRADITIONAL LONG TERM CARE

Traditional long term care is a catch-all term referring to the existing array of services designed to meet the needs of the chronically impaired. Note that the word "system" has deliberately not been used, for it is often the lack of systems that has created the problems motivating the development of alternative demonstrations. To many, long term care has been synonymous with skilled nursing institutional care, but this interpretation obviously is not taken by the community-based demonstrations that have looked at individuals with varying types and degrees of chronic care needs. While the

Rick T. Zawadski is Research Director, On Lok Senior Health Services, 1455 Bush Street, San Francisco, CA 94109.

problems of the younger impaired are often similar, most of the demonstrations have focused on the older impaired population, and for purposes of convenience this monograph retains that emphasis.

The litany of problems associated with traditional long term care has been eloquently stated elsewhere. Congressional hearings on nursing home abuse have described some of the quality of care concerns, and books, for example, Vladeck's *Unloving Care* (1980) and Moss et al.'s *Too Old, Too Sick, Too Bad* (1977), describe some of the real problems facing the impaired older person today. Instead of repeating the detailed examples and problems, this section summarizes some of the broader concerns of traditional long term care.

Broad Public Concerns

Two broad themes run through the various expressions of public concern relating to existing long term care: (1) high cost and (2) quality of care. Both these problems have been exacerbated by the changing demographics.

In 1900 the average life expectancy in the United States was 47 years of age. Less than 4% of the population was 65 years of age or older. In 1978 almost 11% of the population was 65 years of age or older, and life expectancy had increased to 73 years of age for men (U.S. Census Bureau, 1979). The Congressional Budget Office in 1977 projected this growth rate to continue. With increasing life expectancy and population bulges in the decades ahead, the over-65 proportion of the population is expected to swell to 18% by the year 2000 and 26% by the year 2030 (Panneton & Wesolowski, 1979; U.S. Bureau of the Census, 1979).

More relevant to the problem of long term care is the number of old-old, those individuals over 75 years of age who are more likely to suffer from one or more chronic illnesses and have some functional impairments that prevent them from living fully independent lives (Federal Council on Aging, 1979). Between 1980 and the year 2000, the Congressional Budget Office estimates that this population, the ones likely to be in need of long term care, will triple. These projected demographic changes make concern over long term care cost and quality one of the major challenges confronting our society in the years ahead.

Over the past ten years, the cost of long term care has increased more than three-fold, reflecting both the numbers of people served and demand for services, as well as the cost per service unit. The

Congressional Budget Office has projected that national expenditures for long term care would increase from $18.1-20.4 billion in 1976 and to $63.7-74.5 billion in 1985.

Most of the expenditures for long term care have gone for inpatient services with federal programs footing a large part of that bill. On a national basis, Medicaid has been the prime payor for nursing home care, accounting for 60% of all receipts for those services. For the 65+ population, Medicare is the prime payor for acute inpatient hospital care, with over 80% of all Medicare costs (1976) going for inpatient hospitalization. Much of this hospitalization was related to long term care, either the treatment of chronic medical problems, Medicare reimbursement in an extended care facility or, as is increasingly the case, administratively-approved stays resulting from the lack of alternative long term care services.

What have these billions of dollars bought? Unfortunately, not the high quality of health care that Congress envisioned when guaranteeing entitlement to these services through Medicare and Medicaid legislation. In the almost two decades since these programs were initiated, rapid growth in state and federal public health expenditures has led to increased pressures toward cost containment. These efforts have been especially strong with respect to Medicaid—in some states reimbursement rates for nursing home services have been capped at or below costs. Skilled nursing facilities, especially profitmaking programs, have responded to these cost-pressures by holding tough on salary levels and cutting frills. Many believe this cost-cutting has eroded the quality of care in many nursing homes.

Nursing homes are certainly not all bad. Many are tied into the community—are a part of the community. Some are run by nonprofit organizations who subsidize the programs to maintain a high-quality, stimulating environment for low income aged. More importantly, for some severely impaired individuals nursing home care is the best or only solution. The skilled nursing facility is the most efficient, effective way to provide 24-hour nursing care. However, the institutional environment is not the preferred environment for many aged. While the good skilled nursing facility provides safety with ready access to health services, it also represents a semi-restricted environment. Individuals are moved out of their homes and their communities, away from friends and in some cases families, and often on a long-term, if not permanent, basis. Many people would prefer to live more independently, in their homes and their communities, if some support and services could be provided there.

System Problems

The popular problems of cost and quality have received considerable exposure in discussions of long term care. It must be recognized that problems inherent in the United States' health system as it exists today contribute to the quality and cost of care difficulties. Three such issues have appeared as driving forces for some of the innovative demonstrations: structural fragmentation, lack of integrated mechanisms, and disincentives.

Structural fragmentation. Since services typically have been arranged according to reimbursement mechanisms and grant policies, service fragmentation and duplicate administration are encouraged, rewarded by payment systems based on costs rather than results. Today federal, state and local agencies fund long term care services, sometimes separately, sometimes in combination with each other. At each of these levels, social service and medical service programs are separated by different legislative mandates.

Each of the diverse funding sources has spawned and fostered the development of its own set of diverse service providers. Medicare has stimulated the growth of acute medical services through providing major support to hospitals and medical specialists. Medicaid, on the other hand, was legislatively-mandated to guarantee medical care to the poor in our society. Social service and aging programs, e.g., Title XX of the Social Security Act and Titles III and V of the Older Americans Act, fund another set of services, including meals, transportation, senior centers, board and care facilities. And the Department of Housing and Urban Development plays still another role, that is, meeting the housing needs of a portion of the aged and disabled populations.

In a typical community, long term care for dependent adults is available through a number of discrete service providers: acute care hospitals, skilled nursing facilities, home health agencies, day health programs, to name but a few. This fragmentation produces service overlaps, unnecessary duplication in administration, and discontinuity in service response, resulting in less than adequate care for the frail elderly and disabled and unnecessarily high long term care costs.

Adults in need of long term care are rarely able to avoid institutions unless a wide range of supportive medical and social services are readily available. Those capable of remaining in their neighborhoods with only one service are exceptions; yet categorical funding is, by authority and purpose, usually designed to support single services rather than complete systems. Where the need does not fit the category, the frail adult is forced to do without. These gaps are often self-defeating. Without usable transportation, for example, many cannot get medical care in a timely and appropriate way. The result is usually a steady deterioration, ultimately leading to more extensive and costly medical care when care is finally obtained. In a similar way, income maintenance designed to support a wholesome diet may be wasted if meals are not prepared and supervised. With categorical funding sources supporting separate services, an impaired adult often gets what is available rather than what is needed.

With fragmented service providers, some needs may also go unmet. For example, a home health agency cannot meet individual needs for socialization while a pure day health center cannot provide the supportive in-home services. Instead of receiving both as needed, a frail older person must often make the choice of which help to seek or take on the difficulties of dealing with multiple, overlapping agencies. However, simply dealing with multiple providers is itself more than many persons can endure. Relating to many different agencies and individuals and retelling the problems over and over again is an unnecessary burden for the already frail for whom stresses should be alleviated, not increased by the service provider.

Changes in level of care present other problems. The discharge worker in a hospital may recommend in-home follow-up services, but there is no way to guarantee that those services will be delivered or that continuity from the hospital will be maintained. As providers overlap without coordination, they end up repeating or working contrary to each others' objectives. For example, a home health aide may continue to provide meals and personal care after an individual has been rehabilitated to do this for himself.

In addition to all the fragmentation of services that exists across providers, some providers further fragment their services by distinguishing levels or "unbundling" component services. For example, there is often a different basic rate (that is, a "private pay" rate, a "Medicare" rate and a "Medicaid" rate) for every unit within a hospital, with a separate bill for each identifiable service unit—down to the box of tissues.

Fragmentation of services also results in high administrative costs. Every separately billable service also must be separately authorized and separately recorded. When multiple service providers are involved, they must repeat some of the same assessments, imposing an unnecessary cost as well as an added load on the older person.

One may argue that there are good reasons for funding medical care from different pools which reflect federal versus state responsibilities and differences in entitlements. Medicare, for example, is a national, self-supporting insurance program, while Medicaid is federal-state funded from general revenues. But in this battle to differentiate funding responsibility, the needs of the older person have been overlooked. While the impaired older person may have multiple and competing entitlements, his or her needs are interrelated. Today, ironically, services are structured better to meet the needs of the reimbursement agency than the individual in need.

Interestingly, one of the arguments for establishing the Health Care Financing Administration was that if Medicare and Medicaid reimbursement were integrated, the administrative savings would cover the copayment and coinsurance costs now required under Medicare. Unfortunately, eight years later, those reimbursement programs are still effectively separate and those administrative cost savings are yet to be achieved.

Lack of integrating mechanisms. Few of us are trained in the intricacies of health and social service entitlements and procedures. With the large number of fragmented services available, the older impaired person often needs help in sorting out the bewildering array of options, costs and requirements.

One who needs long term care typically suffers from multiple, interrelated chronic problems: medical problems that need ongoing attention, functional impairments that prevent full independence, and often a degree of cognitive impairment that impedes effective competition for survival resources. In addition, the older person is more likely to have limited income and less than adequate housing as a result. Some are fortunate to have families and friends who provide a safe and supportive environment; more often among persons requiring long term care services such informal support is not available. Taken together, many interrelated services are required: medical care, adaptive housing, nutrition, transportation, assistance in the home, and social support.

Recognizing this complexity, each individual service provider usually has a mechanism for care coordination. In the hospitals and nursing homes, discharge planners serve as this mechanism. In the social service agency, it might be the social work supervisor. However, these coordinators work primarily within their own set of services and often can make only simple arrangements for transition.

Without a mechanism for linking, coordinating and integrating all services, the individual in need of help must make do with what he finds, appropriate or not. Those who choose to remain in the community are in an especially difficult bind. While the nursing home provides a comprehensive package—mixing room and board with nursing and health services within one controlled setting—all of these individual services must be pieced together for the impaired person who remains at home.

Lack of incentives. Most business transactions have implicit checks and balances. A seller offers some goods; a buyer purchases those goods if and when s/he determines the goods are of significant value. Traditional long term health care, unfortunately, does not function as simply or as rationally. In the typical transaction, there are three parties: a service recipient who has a set of needs; a service provider who is willing to provide a number of services; and a service reimbursor—public funding program or insurance company—that pays for the services that are delivered.

In this three-party, fee-for-service system, there is little incentive for cost control. The individual receiving services has little or no responsibility for the cost of those services and is willing to request or accept whatever services are offered or made available. The service provider has an incentive to provide more services, for with higher volume, revenues increase and cost per unit of service goes down. The reimbursement agency, typically uninvolved in the day to day transactions, has only the role of policeman, trying to control the absurdly high costs and/or inappropriate levels of service utilization.

With no incentives bearing on those involved directly in the transaction to control use and cost, the reimbursement agent inevitably becomes the "heavy." In representing the collective good of the consumer, the reimbursor ironically is perceived as the force preventing treatment of the individual. In such a system, utilization controls, relegated to a function of reimbursement limitation, are truly responsive to neither individual needs or cost-control concerns, but are intended only to prevent gross abuse. It is not surprising that costs have grown at alarming rates.

THE DEVELOPMENT OF ALTERNATIVES

The concern of reimbursement agencies and policy makers about costs and the frustration of providers at not being able to give, within the scope of their reimbursement, the services they felt were needed by their clients have stimulated the development of alternatives in long term care over the last quarter of a century.

The alternatives fall into two major categories: (1) single service alternatives; and (2) more holistic system alternatives, that is, programs that cut across traditional services seeking to create a more coherent, integrated service system. The variations reflect to some extent the genesis of the alternatives and the predominance of perspective—reimbursor or provider.

The funding/reimbursement agency, whether a legislative body or the agency mandated to implement those services, has sought to contain, control or reduce costs and looked to new service options, sometimes called "alternatives," as either lower cost services or potential overall-cost reducers. Their cost control concerns usually have been narrow, focusing only on a particular pool of funds. For example, Medicare, seeking to control hospitalization, has had little concern whether or not it increases Medicaid-paid long term care placements.

Service providers and consumers have looked to these new alternatives to alleviate their frustrations regarding the quality of care and the restrictions that care entails. For example, as an alternative to the restrictive environments of the hospital and nursing home, consumers and service providers have advocated the development of community-based services for long term care to enable the person to stay in familiar surroundings and more natural settings while receiving services.

Single Service Responses

At the turn of the century, there was little or no need for long term care services. But medical technology improved, resources became available, medical services became increasingly more sophisticated and generally more available. People lived longer and they came to demand more services. The first option available for caring for the chronically-impaired population, often now referred to as the long term care population, was acute medical care, that is, medical services and hospital care.

Acute medical care. Hospitals became the environment where tools and professional resources could be brought together to meet medical problems. The aged constituted a growing proportion of those requiring medical services, and the impaired aged who could not live independently in the community, but needed long-term chronic care, came to dominate the hospital population.

Medicare legislation in the 1960s guaranteed acute medical care to most people over 65 years of age. By providing a strong reimbursement base for acute medical care, Medicare gave hospitals a steady stream of older people requiring these services. Since Medicare is the primary reimbursor to the over-65 middle class population, it has come under increasing pressure to take responsiblility for long term care service needs.

Skilled nursing facility. The skilled nursing facility was one of the first long term care "alternatives"—that is, an alternative to acute hospitalization. Many hospital residents with chronic care needs did not so much require medical sophistication, as ongoing nursing and supportive services. To segregate this population, that is, move them out of expensive hospital beds into less sophisticated nursing facilities where nursing services could be provided on an ongoing basis at a lower cost and in a more holistic, nurturing environment seemed efficient and desirable. When individuals needed acute care, they would be transferred back to the hospital.

The first long term care environment, the nursing home, remains the only environment that provides room and board, as well as supportive services, in one facility. Various levels of nursing home care have evolved (e.g., extended care facility, intermediate care facility) in different parts of the country, usually reflecting different service packages, patient needs and reimbursement rates. Utilization of this service quickly grew so that today almost 5% of the 65+ population resides in such a facility. The skilled nursing facility remains less expensive than a hospital and, for many people with multiple, interrelated needs, is the most efficient provider of ongoing nursing care services.

Home health services. Like the nursing home, home health services developed as an alternative to the high cost of hospitalization. Home health was first encouraged as a way to reduce the hospital stay by allowing professional services such as nursing and therapy to be delivered on a short-term basis in patient's homes. The cost for these professional services on a per service basis was low relative to hospital stay costs, but still significant. Since these services emanated from the acute care perspective, Medicare reimbursement was available, making them a long term care service option for a large segment of people over 65 years of age.

The major benefit of home health services was the movement

away from institutionalization towards community residence. The home health movement triggered this fundamental philosophical shift.

In-home services. Because home health services were not by themselves a sufficient response to the supportive needs of the older person, less professional in-home services were developed. "In-home services" is a generic term referring to the array of personal care, supportive and homemaker services given to individuals in their own homes. These services are reimbursed through Medicare, Medicaid and social service programs. Depending on the reimbursement source, they may include anything from a personal care provider to 24-hour attendant care. Like home health services, in-home services emphasize the individual's continued residence in the community.

Typically, in-home services involve lower cost service providers—aides and paraprofessionals—who provide a broader array of personal and supportive services. While cost per service unit is lower than when professional service providers are involved, the higher number of units often results in a high cost service program. It is not unusual for heavy in-home service support, for example, to cost more than nursing home care. The one-to-one nature of in-home services makes it inefficient when multiple services and large numbers of service units are required.

Day center services. Unlike home health which developed as a response to acute hospitalization, day center programs developed as an alternative to skilled nursing placement. Day center programs— variously called day care, day hospital, and adult day health programs—receive reimbursement from Medicaid, Medicare, social service programs and private donations. Like home health and in-home services, day health emphasizes de-institutionalization, supporting the older person while residing in his own home in his own community. Instead of delivering services in the home, however, day center programs bring people into a community-based day center where services, meals, transportation, nursing and therapy can be provided more efficiently in group settings.

Billed as an alternative to skilled nursing placement, day center programs have faced much tighter cost comparisons than home health programs. It is not unusual in most parts of the country for a day in a center to be reimbursed at levels below the cost of a nursing home day and even below the cost of one single home health service. Absence of significant, secure reimbursement has limited the growth of day centers and low rates of reimbursement have kept programs from developing more professional services.

Perhaps the most significant contribution made by day center programs has been the fundamental shift away from fee-for-service reimbursement. Unlike home health or in-home services where reimbursement is based on the number of units of service (e.g., a 15-minute home or professional nursing contact), the total package of services delivered in the day health center often has one reimbursement rate, with the unit being a day of services. In California's Medicaid reimbursement of adult day health services, that service day includes all nursing, transportation, meals, personal care, supportive, recreation services and most therapy, regardless of number of services of each type received.

Hospice. Recently, a new service has been legislated for reimbursement through Medicare: the hospice. Hospice refers to the package of services given to dying persons and their families in the last six months of life. While very focused in terms of the clientele served and the time period covered, the hospice service represents potentially even greater consolidation of services than in day health. Providers have fuller freedom over services they may deliver, bound only by a cap on total cost of care. It is too early to assess the implementation of this new program, but it does reflect movement towards greater integration and consolidation of services to reflect more closely the needs of the impaired person.

System Alternatives

In the early-to-middle 1970s, with the greater number of service options available and the resultant confusion, attention shifted towards the integration of services. The focus was on two aspects of service integration: (1) structural integration—the merging of different services and funding sources, e.g., the integration of medical, social and supportive services into a single system; and (2) development of integrating mechanisms, e.g., intake/referral, case management, care coordinators.

Central to all the system alternative projects are *waivers* from one of the federal health programs, i.e., Medicare or Medicaid. Waivers permit deviation or variation from normal reimbursement rules and policies. Depending on the funding source involved, different waiver authorities need to be used, different provisions need to be waived and different procedures are employed to obtain those waivers. For Medicare, Section 222 of Public Law of 93-403 is used to fund demonstration projects. Most of the demonstrations waive Medicare's traditional restrictions on the scope of services covered to include additional services, for example, case management, in-home support or transportation. Applications for Medicare waivers are approved directly by the Health Care Financing Administration.

Two waiver authorities allow expanded Medicaid reimbursement: Section 1115 of the 1974 Medicare Act and Section 1915 of the 1981 Omnibus Reconciliation Act. Each has its own advantages and disadvantages, but generally Medicaid waivers will expand the scope of services to be covered by the reimbursement and expand eligibility. All benefits offered by the state in its Medicaid plan must normally be made available to everyone in that state, unless this statewideness requirement is waived. Because Medicaid is a state-run program, the state must submit any Medicaid waiver request; that is, projects seeking Medicaid reimbursement must first get state approval.

Because of the complexity in receiving these waivers, it is not surprising that most of the projects described in this report are either Medicare or Medicaid waivered. Few have both. This limitation has significant implications for the demonstration project's thrust, for each tends to emphasize its reimbursement source's high-cost service factors. For example, Medicare projects have emphasized hospital control; Medicaid projects, nursing home utilization.

Apart from the issue of reimbursement, the models that have emerged among the system alternative demonstrations are now only beginning to be differentiated. Most of these demonstration projects have had a method of integrating services, either structurally or operationally, and the freedom to provide and, in some cases, create new services to fill the gaps in the existing service system.

Two basic systems-approach models can be distinguished although none of the demonstration projects falls neatly into either of these categories. The models are: (1) the brokerage model; and (2) the consolidated direct service model.

Brokerage model. Brokerage models rest upon the premise that existing community-based services can provide an alternative to individuals in need of long term care, if help can be given in finding and arranging appropriate services. Thus, a number of programs have sprung up to coordinate services via case managers or case management teams. Typically, these demonstrations have been initiated by home health agencies or consortiums of community service providers. Often the case manager or case management team is independent of any direct service provider, but uses all of them, primarily providing the necessary coordination.

A case manager, usually a social worker or nurse, visits the individual, provides a summary assessment and determines that person's needs, then, often in consultation with other professional members of a multidisciplinary team, structures the most appropriate service package. The case manager then arranges for and, in many cases, authorizes reimbursement for services delivered by the different providers. To review progress and changes in needs the case manager continues to work with the client and revises the service plan as conditions require.

Triage in Connecticut was probably the most widely-known example of the brokerage model applied to long term care. Other projects include Project OPEN in San Francisco, MSSP in California, and more recently, the National Long Term Care Channeling Project, a multi-state demonstration. Projects vary in degree of services directly provided by the case manager or case management team and vary in the services provided by the parent organization.

A variant of the brokerage model is the "prior-authorization" approach that rests upon the premise that many people going into nursing homes do not require that level of care. Inappropriate nursing home placement occurs either because of lack of alternative services to meet the specific needs or inability to coordinate with these appropriate alternative services. A number of Medicaid-funded projects were therefore developed that had: (1) a review team to assess each person referred for long term care placement, determine the individual's needs and define the services best suited to meet those needs; and (2) authority to reimburse for a collection of non-institutional long term care services, such as home health services and day care services, as more cost-effective alternatives.

Monroe County's Project ACCESS (New York), Georgia's Alternative Health Service project, and South Carolina's Community Long Term Care demonstration are all variants of the prior-authorization approach. In most cases, the screening team functions as part of a public human service agency and has primarily a review function. Projects vary in the amount of direct contact they have with clients. Most control reimbursement for their range of services, but vary in the number of services included in the program and the degree of ongoing client monitoring. Usually these are areawide in scope.

Consolidated direct service model. Unlike the brokerage model which provides case management and coordination of services, the consolidated direct-service model directly responds to a spectrum of needs by delivering services, usually through its own programs. Typically in a consolidated model, a single pool of funds is established to combine diverse funding sources, and payment is made for all services, whether medical, rehabilitative, social supportive or recreational, as a total package rather than on the discrete fee-for-service basis. The participating funding sources have no control over individual services. Of the three, the provider in the consolidated model has the most freedom over the delivery of services and the creation of new services, that is, the greatest ability to respond to individual needs without reimbursement constraints. When the provider is also at financial risk as is sometimes the case, there is a direct cost control responsibility, that is, a built-in incentive.

The best known example of a consolidated model is in the acute care arena, the Health Maintenance Organization (HMO). Recent demonstrations have begun to focus HMOs on the older population, whom HMOs frequently have underserved. Another recent idea, the Social/Health Maintenance Organization or S/HMO, goes beyond the HMO in terms of integrating medical and social services into a single consolidated service package for the general (that is, not long term care specific) 65+ population. In this volume, examples of the consolidated model include On Lok's Community Care Organization for Dependent Adults and Metropolitan Jewish Geriatric Center's site for the Nursing Home Without Walls project.

CONCLUSION

This chapter began by tracing the problems that motivated the development of community-based long term care alternatives. Behind the oft-cited difficulties of cost and quality of care were systematic problems, namely fragmentation, lack of integration mechanisms and lack of incentives. Seeking more appropriate care alternatives is not a new phenomenon—the nursing home itself came to be as an alternative to costly acute hospital care. Single service alternatives have caused new thinking on: *where* care may be provided (that is, in the home as well as in the institution); *who* should provide care (that is, paraprofessionals as well as health professionals); *how* care should be provided (that is, in group settings in the community as well as one-on-one in the home) and how care should be *paid for* (that is, fee-for-service versus a capitation rate for a package of services). In contrast to these single service approaches, the demonstrations under scrutiny in this monograph are system alternatives and are specifically concerned with the integration of services. Finally, these system alternative demonstrations are too new to be differentiated fully but two general types or models have emerged (the brokerage and the consolidated). With this historical and conceptual framework in mind, the projects themselves can be examined.

REFERENCES

Federal Council on the Aging. *Public policy and the frail elderly* (DHEW Publication No. (OHDS) 79-20959). Washington D.C.: U.S. Government Printing Office, 1979.

Moss, F. E., & Halamandaris, V. J. *Too old, too sick, too bad.* Germantown, Maryland: Aspen Systems Corp., 1977.

Panneton, P. E., & Wesolowski, E. F. Current and future needs in geriatric education. *Public Health Reports*, 1979, *94*.

U.S. Bureau of the Census. *Social and economic characteristics of the older population of 1978.* Washington, D.C.: U.S. Government Printing Office, 1979.

U.S. Congressional Budget Office. *Long term care for the elderly and disabled.* Washington, D.C.: Author, 1977.

Vladeck, B. *Unloving care.* New Jersey: Basic Books, 1980.

PART II

THE LONG TERM CARE DEMONSTRATIONS

Introduction

In this section, eight long term health care demonstration projects describe in their own words their programs and share some of the lessons they learned and recommendations they have as they relate to community-based long term care. The eight projects all represent comprehensive coordinated community-based models of long term care.

As an introduction to the eight projects, this section describes: (1) what is meant by "comprehensive, coordinated community-based system of long term care"; (2) some of the criteria for project inclusion; and (3) a description of the format each project was asked to adhere to.

WHAT DO WE MEAN BY COMPREHENSIVE COORDINATED COMMUNITY-BASED SYSTEM OF LONG TERM CARE?

"Comprehensive" means that each of the demonstration projects integrates within its demonstration some medical, social and supportive services. "Coordinated" means that each project uses some method, for example, case management or direct service delivery, to bring together the services in a manner that best meets the needs of the individual. "Community-based" means that each of the demonstrations focuses on community services as a means of delaying or reducing institutional stays. "System" refers to the deliberate attempt on the part of each project to establish procedures for assessment, care coordination and reimbursement that integrate the diverse services needed by the impaired older person into a more rational integrated system. Finally, by the phrase "long term care," it is meant that these projects focus on those individuals who have one or more impairments that put them in need of continuing or chronic health care and supportive services.

CRITERIA FOR PROJECT SELECTION

Many of the projects included in this monograph are well-known, having been talked about in other places. Some may be unfamiliar for they are just now reporting their first returns. In general, projects were selected for inclusion because they represented interesting models of community-based long term care and had important lessons to share with others seeking to develop similar programs. More specifically, to obtain an array of projects that together presented a picture of current developments in community-based long term care, projects had to meet four minimal criteria.

1. *Health reimbursement demonstrations.* Each of the models received reimbursement through at least one of the federal health care reimbursement programs, i.e., Medicare or Medicaid.
2. *Expanded community-based services.* Each of the demonstration projects had to offer or provide access to expanded community-based services. In most cases, these services were provided through waivers allowing coverage by their respective funding source of a broader scope of services.
3. *Service coordination.* Each of the projects had to provide some mechanism for service coordination, whether it be prior authorization screening or referral, case management, or direct service delivery.
4. *Operational with data.* Each project had to be operational—beyond the planning stage and surviving in some form—and to have some data to describe the population, services and costs of their programs; ideally data would also be available to assess the project's impact over time.

In selecting the project chapter authors, an effort was made to identify the primary people involved in the development of those programs. When a program was a statewide program with local sites, an attempt was made to involve persons at both the state and local service provider levels.

PROJECT DESCRIPTION FORMAT

To meet the dual objectives of consistent project description and exploration of critical issues, each of the projects was requested to follow a prescribed format for its chapter. To assist the reader in

362.16 C737m
C.1

looking across projects, each set of authors was asked to include in the first half of the chapter the following sections in this order:

1. *Overview:* a brief synopsis of the project, its development and present status.
2. *Project Origin and Objectives:* the impetus or motivation for the project and the objectives it was to achieve; a brief description of the organizational structure and auspices under which the program operated; and a brief history describing the program's development.
3. *Population Served:* the population the project was intended to serve (target population), the admission requirements to the project, time frames of the program, the number of people served, and summary demographic and functional status data describing that population.
4. *Services:* the services offered by or included in the project, with a special emphasis on the methods or procedures for coordinating or integrating the services.
5. *Funding:* the funding source or sources, with a description of the waivers received in order to obtain that reimbursement; a description of the method of reimbursement, e.g., perspective reimbursement or fee-for-service, and the services that are included in project costs; and a description of the approaches used for cost containment.
6. *Research Design:* the design used for that project, instrumentation, comparison samples and data collection procedures.
7. *Summary of Findings:* the major findings of the research project, especially those focusing on cost and effectiveness impacts.
8. *Lessons Learned:* some of the lessons they learned through their project (based on the implementation and operation experience as well as the interpretation of research findings).

In addition to the common elements in the first half of each chapter, the authors were asked to identify and discuss one of the issues they had to confront or conclusions they had reached in developing their system. The idea, here, was to present insights not usually available in print—important practical and policy issues discovered in the course of real-world program experience. Discussion topics ranged broadly from the importance of targetting the program to the frail to a very frank discussion of life-after-demonstration, that is, what happens to programs when the demonstration ends. Taken together, the reader will find the discussion sections in Part II provide a fresh, thoughtful survey of the major issues confronting community-based long term care today.

Chapter 2

Five Years of ACCESS: What Have We Learned?

Gerald M. Eggert, PhD,
Belinda S. Brodows, MSHyg, MA

OVERVIEW

ACCESS is the case management unit of the Monroe County Long Term Care Program, Inc. (MCLTCP, Inc.), in Rochester, New York. MCLTCP, Inc. began in 1975 as a Section 1115, Health Care Financing Administration (HCFA) demonstration project to develop a community-wide population-based model for the organization, delivery and financing of long term care for the adult disabled and aged. While designing a system that would be more cost effective and of better quality than the existing system, ACCESS set out to demonstrate the feasibility and utility of a freestanding community-based organization for planning and managing long term-care. ACCESS (Assessment for Community Care Services) is the model that evolved.

ACCESS began operating in late 1977 and has been serving the needs of the chronically ill and elderly for over five years. Through the program, increasing numbers of people have received Medicare and Medicaid-reimbursed home care services and nursing home care instead of more costly and inappropriate hospital care.

ACCESS differs from other long term care demonstrations in that it: (1) provides system-wide intervention designed to reduce inappropriate use of acute and long term care institutions; (2) controls

Gerald M. Eggert is Executive Director and Belinda S. Brodows is Deputy Director at the Monroe County Long Term Care Program, Inc., Rochester, New York.

Questions may be directed to Gerald M. Eggert, PhD, Executive Director, Monroe County Long Term Care Program, Inc., Plymouth Park West, 55 Troup Street, Rochester, NY 14608.

27

both Medicaid and Medicare payment approval for long term care; (3) stresses comprehensive, pre-admission assessment but does not provide assessment or other long term care services directly to clients; (4) provides access to expanded Medicaid and Medicare services; and (5) waives Medicaid financial eligibility requirements for the purpose of comprehensive assessment and case management.

ACCESS appears to have reduced the use of acute hospitals and nursing homes through the substitution of appropriate institutional and non-institutional services. Its assessment and service planning approach is backed with the authority to approve public payment for recommended long term care services. Until October 1982 ACCESS had responsibility for Medicaid eligible clients only; with a Section 222 HCFA demonstration grant ACCESS has begun to approve Medicare extended care expenditures for Medicare beneficiaries as well.

PROJECT ORIGIN AND OBJECTIVES

MCLTCP, Inc., is a freestanding, nonprofit organization governed by a board made up of equal numbers of consumers, health professionals (providers) and public officials. The organization developed in response to major national, state and local issues in the long term care field. Its beginnings can be traced to an April 1974 meeting of state and Rochester area officials convened to discuss the problems associated with increasing long term care expenditures. Out of this meeting came a deluge of ideas, a matrix of problems and solutions and a draft for a demonstration grant proposal. More specifically, the establishment and incorporation of MCLTCP, Inc. in 1976 was a result of a joint effort undertaken by the New York State Department of Social Services (NYDSS) and Monroe County, a community at the forefront of long term care improvement efforts for more than 25 years.

The original program was funded by a grant from the federal government to the NYDSS under Section 1115 of the Social Security Act. NYDSS, in turn, contracted with MCLTCP, Inc. By October 1976, the ACCESS program model had been accepted by the MCLTCP, Inc. Board. However, implementing the program required additional state and local initiatives. These included: state legislation passed in 1977 to enable New York State to pay for its share of the Medicaid waiver services; a Memorandum of Understanding with the New York State Health Department to establish

Medicaid reimbursement schedules for assessment and waiver services; to substitute local pre-admission assessment and utilization review forms for state forms; a contract with the Monroe County Department of Social Services that had to be approved by the Monroe County Legislature to transfer Medicaid payment approval to ACCESS; and informal working agreements with more than 60 community planning and provider groups, including the Monroe County Medical Society, eight hospital discharge planning units and the hospital association, 15 home health agencies, 30 long term care facilities and their association, and the Genesee Region Professional Standards Review Organization.

ACCESS began program operations December 15, 1977, with full implementation completed by June 1978. Its specific objectives were:

- To encourage persons needing long term care to choose home care in preference to institutionalization when it is an appropriate alternative and less costly;
- To provide coordination and continuity of case management for long term care clients;
- To improve long term care assessment and review procedures;
- To collect data about the needs, service utilization, and appropriateness of placement of persons requiring long term care to facilitate future planning and evaluation for clients;
- To minimize inappropriate utilization of long term care resources;
- To reduce the number of Monroe County residents who are in acute care hospital beds beyond medical necessity while they await placement in a long term care facility;
- To reduce Monroe County residents' occupancy of long term care institutions through appropriate use of non-institutional alternatives; and
- To reduce increased Medicaid expenditures for individuals needing long term care (including both expenditures for long term care and for alternate care days in acute care hospitals while inpatients wait for long term care arrangements).

In 1980, the program was awarded a grant under Section 222, Title XI which enabled ACCESS to offer and pay for an expanded package of services for Medicare beneficiaries as well. Through this grant, many clients who formerly were only eligible for payment for assessment and case management services (under a Medicaid waiver of financial eligibility) are now able to receive reimbursed nursing home and home care services as well. The rationale behind expanding both the Medicaid and Medicare service packages was to maximize the availability, desirability and use of alternatives to costly hospital care when acute care was not absolutely necessary. By decreasing the inappropriate use of acute care, the program hoped to reduce the rate of growth of both Medicaid and Medicare expenditures—shifting payments from higher to lower cost types of services (both community and nursing home).

PROJECT CHARACTERISTICS

Population Served

The project is designed to serve adults who, for a variety of reasons, are at risk of needing extended long term care (that is, over 90 days in duration). Any adult in Monroe County who is incapable of self-care, needs social and health services to remain at home, or has a physical or psychosocial handicap that interferes with home functioning is eligible for the pre-admission assessment and care planning process. Further, patients of hospitals and other health facilities who need another form of institutional care or who might be discharged if home services are available are also eligible. Under ACCESS, all admissions to nursing homes must be assessed and certified prior to admission if Medicaid payment is required. Between 1978 and 1982, ACCESS assisted 11,444 persons to receive appropriate long term care services. Of this number, 7,292 (64%) were determined to need skilled level placements.

A summary of demographic and functional status data was not available for the total ACCESS client population. However, such a summary was available (Table 1) for a sample of ACCESS home care clients. The sample consisted of 624 ACCESS clients who: (1) were certified as requiring skilled level placements; (2) received home care services rather than nursing home services; and (3) had received home care services for at least one year (Podgorski and Williams, 1983). Because this sample did not include ACCESS' nursing home clients it may not be representative of the overall ACCESS population.

Table 1

CLIENT CHARACTERISTICS

	%		%
Age		Ambulation	
18-64	15	Needs no assistance	25
65-74	20	Walks with assistance	32
75-84	31	Unable to walk without	43
85+	34	human/other assistance	
(n)	(622)	(n)	(582)
Sex		Bathing	
Male	73	Needs no assistance	15
Female	27	Needs partial assistance	30
(n)	(624)	Needs total assistance	55
		(n)	(581)
Source of Referral		Dressing	
Community	68	Needs no assistance	24
Hospital	32	Needs partial assistance	36
(n)	(624)	Needs total assistance	40
		(n)	(571)
Living Situation		Feeding	
Lives alone	26	Needs no assistance	49
Lives w/ others	74	Needs partial assistance	36
(n)	(624)	Needs total assistance	12
		(n)	(539)
Informal Support			
Yes	36		
No	64		
(n)	(518)a		
Payer			
Medicaid	47		
Non-Medicaid	34		
Conversion to Medicaid	19		
(n)	(624)		

Note. This sample includes only those clients who received home care services. These data were drawn from Podgorski & Williams, 1983.

a "Informal Support" n = 518 because those cases in which the client has no needs or the needs are filled by formal supports are not included.

Service Program

Assessment and case management. ACCESS case managers provide "administrative" case management to clients. All direct services—including assessment services—are provided by community agencies and contracting consultants with which it works. Upon referral, Certified Home Health Agency staff and hospital discharge planners complete the pre-admission assessment on all clients. This same assessment is then used by: (1) hospitals as a transfer document when the patient is discharged to a nursing home or his/her own home; (2) the Community Home Health Agency as the basis for developing its plan of care for the client; and (3) the ACCESS case manager to certify the level of care needed by the client, and as the basis for working with the community health nurse in developing and coordinating appropriate home care plans.

With the evaluator, the case manager develops the care plan to be offered to the client. Every effort is made to arrange the least expensive and yet most appropriate mix of services, staffing and equipment. When the decision is made, the case manager works with the community health nurse, discharge planner, client and family to initiate the plan, whether it be home care or institutional admission.

The case manager, under supervision of the Medical Director, assures that services being provided are appropriate by certifying the medical necessity for long term care services for both Medicaid and Medicare program participants. For Medicaid recipients, the case manager may approve institutional placement or home care services up to 75% of their equivalent institutional costs; and an on-site representative from the Monroe County Department of Social Services can approve plans from 75% to 110%. If home care costs exceed 110% of the appropriate level of institutional care, the case manager may submit the plan for consideration to the Monroe County Department of Social Services.

Available services. Under ACCESS, all Medicaid services available in New York State are offered including nursing home care; home nursing and home health aide services; medical equipment and supplies; physical therapy; speech therapy; personal care; medical transportation. Under 1115 waivers, pre-admission assessment and case management services are available in addition to friendly visiting, heavy chore, respite care, housing assistance, moving assistance, social transportation, housing improvement, and adult foster family care.

Under the 222 waivers (ACCESS:Medicare), expanded home health services e.g., an additional 100 days, with up to 24 hours a day of service, are provided, as well as 100 days of nursing home care and waiver of the three-day prior hospital stay. These benefits are provided in addition to and without affecting an individual's regular Medicare benefits. A "sudden decline" provision makes

ACCESS:Medicare benefits available to a nursing home patient who experiences a worsening of condition which might require admission to an acute hospital. To prevent this hospitalization, ACCESS will reimburse the nursing home for a nursing evaluation and the attending physician for a complete medical workup with all diagnostic tests and procedures. When increased physician intervention enables the patient to remain in the nursing home safely, ACCESS:Medicare will pay for daily physician visits to the patient in the nursing home. At the same time, the nursing home can authorize up to 14 days of ACCESS:Medicare coverage and payment if the assessment and physician workup indicate that the patient can be cared for in the nursing home and meets the ACCESS: Medicare medical eligibility requirements. In addition, a more relaxed definition of "skilled care" is used allowing the inclusion of individuals needing multiple unskilled services with daily skilled management and some individuals with suddenly occurring mental health problems.

Funding and Financing Mechanism

The administrative aspects of the program have been funded through Section 1115 (1975-1980) and Section 222 since 1980. A grant from the Administration on Aging (1977-1980) helped delineate the case manager role, expand outreach efforts and increase the availability of non-institutional and often non-Medicaid reimbursable resources such as nutrition programs and subsidized housing.

Case management costs for Monroe County Medicaid recipients are reimbursed through regular county Medicaid funds through a contract between Monroe County and ACCESS because ACCESS performs functions which otherwise would be performed by the Monroe County Department of Social Services. The cost of 1115 waivered services is paid in the usual manner through a 50% federal, 25% state and 25% local match. Case management costs for the Medicare clients as well as costs associated with ACCESS: Medicare services are covered through the Medicare Trust Fund. ACCESS approves all payment for services and then submits this information to Medicaid and Medicare for actual payment.

Waivers. In addition to expanding covered services, the 1115 waivers have relaxed Medicaid financial eligibility requirements for the purpose of reimbursing assessment and case management services for non-Medicaids in an attempt to deter their premature and inappropriate institutional admission. A recent survey showed that 35% of those who received assessment services under this waiver indicated the assessment changed their minds about entering a nursing home (MCLTC, Inc., June 1983).

Cost control mechanisms. Both Medicare and Medicaid have traditionally been fee-for-service programs. While ACCESS has administered both programs on this basis, some alternative methods of reimbursement for home health and nursing home services have been developed. Instead of payment for a personal care aide on an hourly per-client basis, ACCESS staff has worked with the Monroe County Department of Social Services to demonstrate that one salaried aide can more efficiently serve several patients on a daily basis (Monroe County Office of Aging, 1981). This concept has proven to be particularly cost effective in high-rise housing and in densely populated neighborhoods where many disabled Medicaid recipients live.

Under ACCESS:Medicare, higher reimbursement rates for skilled nursing facilities (SNFs) are intended to result in shorter hospital stays, quicker readmissions to nursing homes of hospitalized patients, use of hospitalization by nursing homes only when unavoidable, and thus reductions in both Medicare and Medicaid hospital payments.

The ACCESS:Medicare nursing home rate was designed to be prospective and fixed. To date, most SNFs have been reluctant to accept a prospective rate, which cannot be adjusted, to serve patients whose needs may require more costly methods of care than the historic Medicare admissions on which the rate was based. However, those ten facilities for which ACCESS:Medicare was able to promulgate a moderately high prospective rate (up to 15% greater than their Medicaid rate), have been cooperative participants in the ACCESS:Medicare program.

RESEARCH AND EVALUATION

Research Design

To test the impact of the 1115 ACCESS model on the Medicaid program, a three-year evaluation was developed and performed by MACRO Systems, Inc. (1978, 1979, 1980). In the initial phases of the evaluation, the NYSDSS selected six comparison counties in New York State on the basis of their similarity to Monroe County.

Using the county as the unit of analysis, countywide measures were obtained to examine differential impacts on Medicaid long term care costs across counties over pre-/post-ACCESS periods using a non-equivalent control group design (Campbell & Stanley, 1963). Because MCLTCP, Inc. is a systems intervention and intends to impact on the countywide long term care system, this design was deemed most appropriate.

For Monroe and the comparison counties, time-series data were analyzed related to: (1) hospital back-up patients and days, using available data from the Rochester Regional Hospital Association and the Genesee Region Professional Standards Review Organization (GRPSRO); and (2) Medicaid expenditures per beneficiary and by type of service, using data supplied to the New York State Department of Social Services by county departments of social services. Because the program was fully in place by March 1978, this date was considered the point of "ACCESS implementation" for the time-series analysis. The evaluation addressed the accomplishment of the MCLTCP, Inc. Board's previously stated objectives.

With the implementation of ACCESS:Medicare, a new evaluation contractor was hired by HCFA to look at the combined Medicaid and Medicare programs. To establish a stronger link between ACCESS implementation and the use and cost of acute and long term care services, a randomly selected cohort of persons applying for Medicare long term care benefits under ACCESS is being tracked, along with control cohorts in two other counties where no comparable long term care program exists. Results of the 1115 evaluation will be reported here in addition to available information from the Medicare 222 program that began in November, 1982.

Research Findings

Disposition. Results from 1978-1982 (Table 2) show that referral source may be an important factor in the disposition of SNF level clients. Of those referred by the community ($n = 2803$), 91% went home compared to only 44% of those referred by a hospital ($n = 4373$). Breaking this down by year in Table 2, increasing proportions of clients who qualify for SNF care admission are receiving home care services as opposed to nursing home services.

ACCESS also may have impacted the rate of nursing home admission for non-Medicaid referrals. Based on very preliminary data (Table 3) for the first five months of the ACCESS:Medicare program, this expanded home benefit appears to be successful. During

Table 2

SKILLED LEVEL PLACEMENTS FOR COMMUNITY REFERRALS
(1978 - 1982)

| | Home | | Nursing Home | |
	Medicaid	Non-Medicaid	Medicaid	Non-Medicaid
1978	284 (88%)	197 (75%)	37 (12%)	67 (25%)
1979	188 (96%)	286 (89%)	8 (4%)	37 (11%)
1980	147 (97%)	424 (91%)	4 (3%)	43 (9%)
1981	165 (98%)	392 (92%)	4 (2%)	32 (8%)
1982	169 (98%)	296 (94%)	3 (2%)	20 (6%)
Total	953 (94%)	1595 (88%)	56 (6%)	199 (12%)
	2548 (91%)		255 (9%)	2803 (100%)

SKILLED LEVEL PLACEMENTS FROM HOSPITALS
(1978 - 1982)

| | Home | | Nursing Home | |
	Medicaid	Non-Medicaid	Medicaid	Non-Medicaid
1978	102 (35%)	92 (19%)	193 (65%)	388 (81%)
1979	229 (57%)	82 (20%)	174 (43%)	330 (80%)
1980	266 (57%)	134 (27%)	203 (43%)	367 (73%)
1981	368 (68%)	144 (26%)	172 (32%)	415 (74%)
1982	452 (70%)	60 (27%)	198 (30%)	161 (73%)
Total	1417 (64%)	512 (24%)	783 (36%)	1661 (76%)
	1929 (44%)		2444 (56%)	4373 (100%)
Total Both Groups	2370 (74%)	2107 (53%)	839 (26%)	1860 (47%)

Table 3

ACCESS: MEDICARE RESOLUTIONS
(October 30, 1982 - March, 1983)

Referral Source	Dispositions						Grand Total
	Home		Nursing Home		Total		
	Medicaid	Private Pay	Medicaid	Private Pay	Medicaid	Private Pay	
Community	29 (97%)	127 (93%)	1 (3%)	9 (7%)	30 (18%)	136 (82%)	166
	156 (95%)		10 (5%)				
Hospital	53 (32%)	198 (60%)	113 (68%)	124 (40%)	166 (33%)	332 (67%)	498
	251 (51%)		237 (48%)				

this time, 60% of the private-pay ACCESS:Medicare clients went home from hospitals instead of to nursing homes compared to 24% of the private-pay clients who went home from hospitals from 1978-82 (Table 2).

Traditionally SNFs have been reluctant to accept Medicaid clients because of low reimbursement. As indicated in Table 3, 68% of the Medicaid clients referred from hospitals who are disabled enough to be eligible for ACCESS:Medicare have been admitted to nursing homes, compared to only 30% in 1982 (Table 2). The higher proportion of ACCESS Medicare/Medicaid clients entering nursing homes since October 1982 has been accompanied by a 36% decline in the number (110 to 70) of Medicaid clients backed-up in hospitals awaiting nursing home placement.

The very preliminary results presented in Table 4 (disability scores compared to average SNF history) indicate that ACCESS: Medicare is influencing nursing homes to care for a more disabled population. Disability scores reflect three components, namely, an average mobility score, an activities of daily living score and a psycho-behavioral score. The ACCESS clients who qualify for the special Medicare nursing home rate have an average disability score 24% higher (327 vs. 262) than the average scores of patients who have been admitted (1978-1982) to Monroe County SNFs. Similarly, the disability scores of ACCESS:Medicare enrollees who are readmitted to SNFs (369) or for whom hospital admission has been avoided through the special "sudden decline" benefit (367) are higher than patients readmitted to nursing homes prior to the inception of ACCESS:Medicare (339).

Hospital back-up. Hospital back-up is a term which describes patients who remain in an acute care facility when acute care is not medically necessary because appropriate and less expensive non-acute services are not available. Table 5 presents data on the hospital back-up in Monroe County and comparison counties. As shown, the back-up problem is more severe in the counties where no special long term care program exists (Broome and Onondaga). For Medicare hospital days, back-up days increased from 1978 to 1979 in both these counties, while Medicaid back-up days decreased in one of these counties but increased in the other. A look at the total Federal inpatient hospital days filled by backed-up patients in 1979 showed Monroe to have a less severe problem than the comparison counties.

Per-person Medicaid expenditures. Monroe County, pre- to post-

Table 4

FUNCTIONAL STATUS OF SNF CLIENTS BY REVIEW TYPE[a]

	All Reviews		Admission		Readmission		Continued Stay	
	N	Avg	N	Avg	N	Avg	N	Avg
ACCESS (1978-82)	103,671	321	10,254	262	3,476	339	88,193	328
ACCESS:Medicare (1982-83)	137	354	46	327	27	369	64	367
• "Sudden Declines"	(33)	369)	----------	----------	----------	----------	(33)	369)[b]
• All Other Reviews	(104)	349)	(46)	327)	(27)	369)	(31)	365)[c]

[a]Functional status is a combined measure of Average Mobility, ADL and Psychobehavioral Score, the higher the score the higher the disability.

[b]Includes 4 reassessments of patients granted the "sudden decline" benefit; average score for these patients was 382.

[c]Includes 19 reassessments of patients first admitted under ACCESS:Medicare whose average score was 351, and 12 reassessments of patients admitted under ACCESS:Medicare whose average score was 386.

39

Table 5

HOSPITAL BACK-UP DAYS FOR MONROE, BROOME AND ONONDAGA COUNTIES
FEDERAL PAYORS ONLY: 1978-1979

	Monroe County			Broome County			Onondaga County		
	1978	1979[a]	Change	1978	1979	Change	1978	1979	Change
Medicare Back-up Days	45,744	42,879	-6%	21,648	27,304	+26%	13,801	24,309	+76%
Medicaid Back-up Days	3,578	4,341	+21%	2,616	1,280	-51%	1,057	2,950	+79%

Note. This data was drawn from Price, Ripps & Piltz, 1980.

[a] 1979 Data for Monroe County are suspected to be low.

ACCESS, had a lower percentage increase (20%) in the average per-beneficiary Medicaid expenditures for the aged than any of the six comparison counties over that period (see Table 6).

ACCESS's greatest impact on Medicaid expenditures seems to have occurred during its first year of full-scale operations (rate of increase for Monroe - 20%, six-county weighted average - 39%), although Monroe County's rate of increase was also lower in the second year following implementation (Monroe - 9%, six-county weighted average - 16%). It is likely that Monroe's lesser increase in monthly Medicaid expenditures-per-eligible is due to increased

Table 6

PRE-POST-ACCESS
AVERAGE MEDICAID EXPENDITURES PER BENEFICIARY
PER MONTH FOR AGE 65 AND OVER

	Pre-ACCESS[a]		Post-ACCESS[b]		Percent Increase
	Mean Persons	Cost Per Person	Mean Persons	Cost Per Person	Cost Per Person
County					
Monroe	5,573	$449.41	6,067	$537.87	20%
Comparison Counties					
Albany	2,713	539.97	2,886	679.06	26
Westchester	7,314	558.96	8,009	713.00	28
Broome	2,261	338.98	2,228	463.22	37
Suffolk	7,542	403.06	7,813	570.00	41
Onondaga	4,805	358.56	4,970	514.73	44
Erie	9,306	325.04	8,402	516.10	59
Weighted Average of Comparison	5,657	$415.30	6,729	$577.43	39

Note. This data has been taken from Price, Ripps & Piltz, 1980.

[a]27 months prior to ACCESS Implementation (March, 1978)

[b]24 months following ACCESS Implementation

use of home health care services initiated through ACCESS case management efforts. Costing less, on the average, than comparable institutional services, these home health services are provided to more Medicaid recipients enabling: (1) Monroe's costs to remain relatively more stable than its counterpart counties and (2) Monroe's Medicaid dollars to be distributed across a wider segment of the population.

Medicaid expenditures by long term care service. Countywide Medicaid expenditures were monitored in the seven counties to determine whether institutional cost rate declines were matched by home health care cost rate increases. Four expenditure categories were used for this analysis: (1) public and private acute hospital inpatient care; (2) public and private nursing home care (SNF); (3) public and private health related (ICF) facilities; and (4) home care (purchased personal care services, home health aides' services, and nursing service in the home). Since the acute hospital expenditures reflected all hospital days, only 10%-15% of which were for back-up care, the other categories' results were of more interest.

As shown in Table 7, for all four categories combined, Monroe's costs increased about 19% during the pre- to post-ACCESS period. The average cost increase across the comparison counties was 33% and all were higher than Monroe. With respect to nursing home costs, Monroe's also increased the least, 6%, reflecting the slower rate of growth in Medicaid nursing home use in Monroe County over the post ACCESS: Medicaid period. For acute hospital care, Monroe's increase (36%) was about the same as the other six counties' average (37%); however, some of Monroe's increase may have been due to back-up care increases resulting from the closing of 77 nursing home beds in 1979. Monroe's home care costs, as expected, increased more than the average of the other six counties (131% vs. 57%); in fact, only one of the other counties experienced a higher increase than did Monroe.

With caution, it can be estimated that ACCESS saved the public between $5 and $8 million over its first three years. This savings estimate does not consider possible savings to voluntary Medicare and private pay clients from ACCESS case management services nor savings at less than the skilled nursing level of care. The estimate does assume that without ACCESS 20%-30% of those served at home would have backed-up in acute care hospitals and that increases in home-care clients followed a linear trend between annual census points.

Table 7

MEDICAID EXPENDITURES
MONROE AND COMPARISON COUNTIES
PRE-POST ACCESS

	Pre-ACCESS		Post-ACCESS		Change
	Amount	%	Amount	%	
Monroe					
Intermediate Care Facilities	$ 9,952,262	11.2	$12,171,086	11.5	+22.3%
Hospital Services Inpatient	24,454,668	27.5	33,380,742	31.6	+36.5
Nursing Home Care	52,538,246	59.1	55,525,410	52.5	+6.7
Home Health Care	2,016,000	2.3	4,655,000	4.4	+131.0
Total	$88,960,176	100.0	$106,732,238	100.0	+18.9%
Average For Comparison Counties					
Intermediate Care Facilities	$ 9,459,348	10.8	$14,018,966	12.0	+48.2%
Hospital Services Inpatient	30,196,368	34.3	41,357,473	35.5	+37.0
Nursing Home Care	42,784,305	48.7	52,674,000	45.2	+23.1
Home Health Care	5,454,622	6.2	8,577,888	7.3	+57.2
Total	$87,895,643	100.0	$116,628,327	100.0	+32.7%

Note. These data have been taken from Price, Ripps & Piltz, 1980.

[a] Pre-ACCESS Period (1976$_{Q2}$ through 1978$_{Q1}$);

[b] Post-ACCESS Period (1978$_{Q2}$ through 1980$_{Q1}$);

[c] NYSDSS uses the term ICF for Health Related Facilities (HRFs).

LESSONS LEARNED

In implementing the ACCESS program, one of the problems which had to be addressed was the attitudes of clients and service providers towards utilization of long term care services, reimbursement for services, and other administrative issues. Incentives can be placed within the system to change both client and provider behavior so that existing resources are used in a more desirable and cost effective manner. The ACCESS Medicaid program and now ACCESS:Medicare seem to have resulted in alterations in the traditional patterns of acute hospital, nursing home and home care use.

A comprehensive pre-admission assessment, case management and increased post acute benefits have served as the incentives for changing client behavior. Access to information about home care services, available through the ACCESS assessment process, is an important factor in reducing institutionalization. Both the availability of payment for an expanded scope of home care services and difficulty in accessing nursing home beds seemed to influence more Medicaid patients to choose home care over institutional care. In addition, the provision of formal services in the home seems to result in the continued availability of extensive informal supports (Morris, Sherwood & Gutkin, 1981).

Alterations in reimbursement policy can be used to change provider behavior. Because of traditional reimbursement practices, providers often prefer the least disabled individual who can qualify for their level of care. Heavily disabled patients end up spending time in hospitals while they wait for admission to SNF's. The additional reimbursement provided through ACCESS:Medicare has encouraged SNF's to admit some heavily disabled patients, and more quickly readmit them following hospitalization.

In terms of home health services, more flexible benefits were needed because of limited coverage, e.g., no routine aide services for nights and weekends. Perhaps because of limited coverage and availability of home health services prior to ACCESS, service planners often recommended institutionalization over home care. ACCESS waivers removed the barriers to provision of home care services caused by reimbursement requirements and limitations.

Federal policies which are designed to reduce Medicare and/or Medicaid expenditures by reducing benefits in nursing home or home care or by shifting costs from one to the other may, in the end, increase overall expenditures for both programs. ACCESS has shown that by integrating Medicare and Medicaid some of the problems associated with excessive hospital use by both programs can be reduced.

DISCUSSION: MAJOR SERVICE DELIVERY ISSUES IN LONG TERM CARE

In altering traditional patterns of service utilization, ACCESS has had to confront major service delivery issues confronting the long term care field today. These issue areas are: the role of alternatives to institutional care; the responsibility for reimbursement of services; and the organizational and control arrangements for service delivery.

Alternatives

Although there is a clear mandate for the development and provision of alternatives to institutional care (both acute and nursing home) for people who have severe long term care needs, questions remain about the role of these alternative services. Are they simply costly additions to the existing service system or can they be designed to substitute for more expensive acute and long term institutional care? How should services be provided to those who would otherwise enter acute hospitals or nursing homes? Or more subtly, how can one identify those who would linger in acute hospitals for extended stays because nursing homes will not admit them in a timely fashion and for whom home care is not feasible or offered as an option?

The rationale behind ACCESS' expanded Medicaid and Medicare service packages was to maximize the availability, desirability and use of alternatives to costly hospital care when acute care was not absolutely necessary. By decreasing the inappropriate use of acute care, the program hoped to reduce the rate of growth of both Medicaid and Medicare expenditures by shifting payments from higher to lower cost types of services (both community and nursing home).

Has this approach been successful? Results from 1978-1982 have shown increasing proportions of clients who qualify for SNF care admission have either chosen to stay in the community and receive home care services or have returned home from hospitals instead of entering a nursing home.

Reimbursement Source

A major problem for policymakers has been determining who should pay for long term care. The Medicare program, designed as an acute care payment program initially, paid for limited nursing home benefits. The rapid rise in program expenditures, however, resulted in sharp cutbacks so that Medicare now pays for only 2% of nursing home days (1.2% in Monroe County in 1982). Concurrent with cutbacks in the nursing home benefit have been enormous increases in Medicare hospital expenditures. What proportion of these acute care increases result from beneficiaries staying longer in hospitals because they have no guaranteed Medicare payment to a skilled nursing home at discharge? Was the Medicare program fiscally better off when it paid for limited nursing home benefits as a means of containing the growth of the acute benefits? Similarly Medicaid program expenditures have also increased. Since Medicaid is the primary source of payment for long term care, have cutbacks in Medicare payments for nursing home care resulted in increased Medicaid hospital expenditures (by creating a class of Medicaid hard-to-place patients who remain in acute hospitals for extraordinary lengths of stay)?

In the first five years, the ACCESS program focused on serving Medicaid recipients while in the past two years the incorporation of Medicare beneficiaries has been planned and implemented. Why has ACCESS developed a program for both Medicare and Medicaid?

ACCESS uses a systemwide approach to solving the policy issues which have been raised, viewing the health care system components—acute hospital care, long- and short-term skilled nursing facility care and long- and short-term home care—as closely related. For example, a patient cannot be discharged from a hospital if there are no accessible nursing home beds if the patient has no "home" to which to return.

Source of reimbursement is important from a systemwide perspective. Concurrent with the tightening of the Medicare skilled nursing benefit has been an increase in Medicare hospital use (HCFA, 1981).

Since Medicare and Medicaid funds ultimately come from the

same source—the taxpayer—fusing aspects of these two programs makes some sense. With fusion, the advantages of each can be maximized and the inequalities suffered by Medicare beneficiaries, who have little available reimbursable nursing home and home care services, and Medicaid recipients, who have great difficulty being admitted to nursing homes, can be minimized.

This objective of equalizing benefits available to Medicare and Medicaid clients so that both programs can gain from measures to assure cost effectiveness (as opposed to cost shifting) is a major component of ACCESS. The increased accessibility of home health services under ACCESS:Medicare equalized the reimbursement of home care for both Medicare and Medicaid patients. For clients needing nursing home admission the incentives are also more nearly equal. Under ACCESS:Medicare, some SNFs are reimbursed at a daily rate which exceeds their current Medicaid rates, and is closer to their actual cost of caring for the more heavily disabled client.

Organization and Control

Experience gained through demonstration projects has resulted in various organizational and control arrangements. Some programs are provider-based, others community-based, others part of governmental structures. Some provide direct services; others broker through other community agencies which provide services. Some programs authorize payment as well as arrange and manage services while others only manage services. Which organizational efforts are the most desirable from a client's point of view? Which are the most efficient in terms of delivering services? Which are the most acceptable from the perspective of existing providers in the community? Which are the most cost effective?

ACCESS provides no direct services—not even assessment services—to clients. The model was organized as a brokerage system in order to maximize the use of existing community agencies and minimize duplication of efforts. Through ACCESS both payors and multiple providers have come to use the same instrumentation, so paperwork is minimized for all involved.

ACCESS is a freestanding, community-based not-for-profit corporation which operates through contractual relationships with governmental agencies. The rationale behind this approach is that ACCESS, by virtue of its independent status, can objectively determine the level and type of care most appropriate to meet the needs of all its clients.

ACCESS has not only met the needs of its clients, it has been effective in assuring that services are provided in the least restrictive (and least costly) environment. It has a continuing role in assuring appropriate utilization of service through its integration of Medicaid and Medicare benefits.

REFERENCES

Campbell, D. J., & Stanley, J. C. *Experimental and quasi-experimental design for research.* Chicago: Rand McNally College Publishing Co., 1968.

Health Care Financing Administration. *HCFA program statistics of the Medicare and Medicaid data book.* Washington, DC: Author, 1981.

Monroe County Long Term Care Project. *Assessment survey.* Rochester, New York: June 1983.

Monroe County Office For Aging. *High rise personal care homemaker program: (Shared Aide Service: A cost comparison).* Rochester, New York: Author, 1981.

Morris, J. N., Sherwood, S., & Gutkin, C. E. *Meeting the needs of the impaired elderly: The power and resiliency of the informal support system.* Boston: Hebrew Rehabilitation Center for the Aged, November, 1981.

Podgorski, M. S., & Williams, T. F. *Predictors of successful home care plans* (0090-AR-0036). Rochester, New York: University of Rochester, Center on Aging, 1983.

Price, L. C., Piltz, D. M., & Clemans, S. *Evaluation of the Monroe County long term care program.* Silver Spring, MD: Macro Systems Inc., 1978.

Price, L. C., Ripps, H. M., & Piltz, D. M. *Second year evaluation of the Monroe County long term care program.* Silver Spring, MD: Macro Systems Inc., 1979.

Price, L. C., Piltz, D. M., & Clemans, S. *Third year evaluation of the Monroe County long term care program.* Silver Spring, MD: Macro Systems Inc., 1980.

Chapter 3

The Georgia Alternative Health Services Project: Cost-Effectiveness Depends on Population Selection

Albert Skellie, PhD
Florence Favor, BS
Cynthia Tudor, MA
Richard Strauss, MA

OVERVIEW

Georgia's Alternative Health Services (AHS) Project was designed to test the cost-effectiveness of a comprehensive system of community-based long term care services. Services were offered, on a voluntary basis, to elderly Medicaid recipients as an alternative to institutional care.

The project, through contractual arrangements with providers, offered a range of community-based long term care services intended to prevent unnecessary or premature nursing home placement. In addition to regular Medicaid-reimbursed services, three

Albert Skellie and Florence Favor are affiliated with the Georgia Department of Medical Assistance, Atlanta. Cynthia Tudor is a doctoral candidate at Johns Hopkins University and Richard Strauss is with Whittaker Medicus, San Diego, CA.

This project was funded in part by USDHHS Health Care Financing Administration Grant No. 11-P-90334/4-05 administered by the Georgia Department of Medical Assistance. The views expressed in this paper are those of the authors, and no official endorsements by the Georgia Department of Medical Assistance or the USDHHS Health Care Financing Administration are intended or should be inferred. Questions may be directed to Albert Skellie, Alternative Health Systems, Georgia Department of Medical Assistance, 2 Martin Luther King, Jr. Drive, S.E., Atlanta, GA 30334.

The authors gratefully acknowledge review of and comment on the project's *Final Report,* from which much of this paper is derived, by Ruth Coan, Lyman Dennis, and Leslie Saber.

49

categories of services were offered: Alternative Living Services, Adult Day Rehabilitation and Home Delivered Services. The project screened and assessed potential clients to determine eligibility and appropriateness of community-based services. The project, funded by the Health Care Financing Administration and administered by the Georgia Department of Medical Assistance, began in July 1976 and offered services as a demonstration through June 1980.

At the conclusion of the demonstration period, project services continued to be offered through the state Medicaid program. At present, the AHS program is expanding statewide, and it offers services to Medicaid clients through waivers under section 2176 of the Omnibus Budget Reconciliation Act of 1981. A Community Care for the Elderly Act passed by the Georgia General Assembly in the 1982 session mandates statewide assessment for community-based long term care of all applicants for Medicaid-reimbursed nursing home care by July 1985.

PROJECT ORIGIN AND OBJECTIVES

In response to a staff member's conviction that there must be a cost-effective alternative to nursing home care, former Governor George Busbee initiated the development of a grant proposal for a study of community-based health services. The approved grant funded the AHS Project.

The initial grant application proposed three principal research objectives related to the utilization, cost, and effectiveness of alternative services. The project was to investigate whether:

• Premature or unnecessary nursing home placements could be prevented and the growth in Medicaid-financed nursing home populations controlled;
• Less expensive alternatives to nursing home care were possible and could be implemented; and
• More effective services could be provided by a system of comprehensive alternative care arrangements than were then being provided for patients who had the capacity to be self-sufficient.

As the demonstration progressed, it became clear that additional research questions should also be addressed, namely: "For whom, under what circumstances, and with what package of services can community-based long term care be expected to be cost-effective?''

The Georgia Department of Medical Assistance, the agency responsible for all aspects of the Medicaid program in Georgia, administered the AHS project. Between October 1976 and June 1980, the project negotiated contracts with 20 service providers—13 existing health or social service organizations and seven newly developed for the project. Whenever feasible, the project coordinated its services with those of existing programs. For example, to develop homemaker services, the project either contracted directly or encouraged sub-contracting with agencies already delivering these services through other funding sources (e.g., Title III of the Older Americans Act or Title XX of the Social Security Act). Another example was the use of Community Mental Health Agencies as providers of Alternative Living Services.

Finally, the project maintained close ties with the Georgia Department of Human Resources, Division of Family and Children Services (DFACS). Many referrals came through the county DFACS office where AHS intake caseworkers were housed.

PROJECT CHARACTERISTICS

Population Served

In order to be eligible for AHS services, clients were required to be Medicaid-eligible, at least 50 years of age, and certified as eligible for nursing home care. Participants lived in a 17-county target area, including two of the ten Georgia Department of Human Resources service districts. One district was predominantly urban—the seven counties surrounding and including Atlanta (about 1.8 million people). The other district consisted of the ten predominantly rural counties surrounding and including Athens (about 200,000 people).

Table 1 presents the characteristics at the time of enrollment of AHS clients for whom up to 24 months of evaluation data are available. The "E" (experimental) columns show the characteristics of individuals referred to providers for project services; "C" columns describe randomly assigned controls (a description of E and C groups is provided later in this chapter). A total of 444 experimental and 135 control group members were followed for up to 24 months. Findings based on this "24-month sample" will be emphasized in

Table 1

BASELINE CLIENT CHARACTERISTICS BY GROUP

	Experimental %	Control %
Age		
50-59	8	10
60-69	21	13
70-79	33	33
80-89	30	39
90 & Over	8	5
(n)	(442)	(134)
Sex		
Male	28	27
Female	72	73
(n)	(444)	(135)
District		
Atlanta	62	69
Athens	38	31
(n)	(444)	(135)
Race		
White	50	53
Black	50	46
Other	0	1
(n)	(444)	(135)
Marital Status		
Married	25	30
Widowed, Separated, Divorced	65	65
Single	10	5
(n)	(439)	(135)
Referrer		
Self, Family, Friends	22	25
Physician, Hospital,		
Nursing Home	16	18
DFACS	40	38
Other	22	19
(n)	(442)	(134)
Initial Residence		
Private or Boarding Home	92	90
Other	8	11
(n)	(438)	(133)

Table 1 (cont'd)

	Experimental %	Control %
Others at Residence		
Alone	31	27
With Spouse	24	28
With Others	45	45
(n)	(438)	(133)
Service Recommendation		
ALS	3	7
ADR	22	20
HDS	38	36
HDS/ADR	23	22
Other	15	16
(n)	(441)	(135)
Client Service Preference		
ALS	6	11
ADR	22	21
HDS	46	47
HDS/ADR	20	14
Other	7	7
(n)	(436)	(131)
GMCF Recommendation		
Intermediate Care	88	91
Skilled Nursing	12	8
Other	0	1
(n)	(381)	(110)
Number of Diagnoses		
1-3	65	70
4-6	32	25
7-9	4	5
(n)	(444)	(134)
Primary Diagnosis		
Diabetes	6	10
Cerebrovascular	14	18
Neoplasm	3	6
Heart Disease	12	11
Arthritis	9	10
Hypertension	12	10
Fracture	3	2
Organic Brain Syndrome	2	1
Other	41	32
(n)	(444)	(134)

Table 1 (cont'd)

	Experimental %	Control %
Mental Status		
0-1 Items Missed	35	23
2-3 Items Missed	29	44
4-7 Items Missed	24	24
8-10 Items Missed	12	9
(n)	(373)	(113)[a]
Walking		
No Help	42	43
Cane	17	20
Crutches, Walker	16	13
Personal Assistance	13	9
Does Not Walk	13	16
(n)	(434)	(135)
Activities of Daily Living		
0 (Most Independent)	40	42
1	25	24
2	10	11
3	8	5
4	7	8
5	5	5
6 (Most Dependent)	5	6
(n)	(435)	(132)
Instrumental Activities of Daily Living[b]		
(1-Most Independent:	2.13	2.18
3-Most Dependent) S.D.	.56	.54
(n)	(443)	(135)
Morale		
(1 = Lowest:	1.53	1.53
2 = Highest) S.D.	.33	.30
(n)	(416)	(127)

Note. For clients with 24 months of data. Only significant chi-square values are shown. Raw chi-square values are reported in the table.

[a] $x^2 = 10.86$ $p < .05$ $df = 3$

[b]Represents mean and standard deviation of each group.

this project report. In all, 1,102 experimental and 320 control group clients were enrolled in the project through December 1979.

The majority of project clients were 70 years of age or older, and almost three-quarters were women. The groups contained about equal proportions of Blacks and Whites. About two-thirds of the clients were widowed. Most clients lived with others and most lived in a private house or apartment at the time of enrollment. About two-thirds of the clients lived in the metropolitan Atlanta area.

The Department of Family and Children Services (DFACS) accounted for the largest percentage of referrals, although a substantial proportion were referred by family and friends. At the time of initial assessment, clients generally were either dependent on another person or some appliance in order to go outside or walk on level ground, and most were dependent in one or more basic Activities of Daily Living (ADL). Mental status scores (SPMSQ) were concentrated at the upper end of the scale, with most clients missing fewer than four of ten items; on both Instrumental Activities of Daily Living (IADL) and the morale scale, mean scores were about midway between the highest and lowest scores possible. Most clients had from one to three diagnoses, although about one-third had between four and six diagnoses. The most common primary diagnoses were heart disease, hypertension, and cerebrovascular disease.

Services Provided, Screening and Case Management

Prior to the AHS project, few Medicaid reimbursable alternatives to institutional long term care were available. Under Section 1115 Medicaid waivers, services not otherwise available under the Georgia Medicaid program could be offered. Three categories of services were offered, alone or in combination:

> *Alternative Living Services (ALS)*—both personal care services and daily activity supervision in supportive living arrangements (including adult foster care, boarding care, or congregate living) for clients unable to function independently in their own homes.
> *Adult Day Rehabilitation (ADR)*—ambulatory health care and health-related supportive services within an adult day care center for clients otherwise able to live independently without 24-hour care.

Home Delivered Services (HDS)—traditional skilled home health services in the client's home along with homemaker services, home delivered meals, and medical appliances and equipment.

Medically-related transportation was available as part of the special services package, with other regular Medicaid reimbursed services available as required. Finally, clients were assisted in locating and utilizing health and health-related services provided through other community-based service agencies.

Screening, placement and case management systems and procedures had to be developed and implemented. The screening and placement system was designed to permit assessment of clients' service needs, to identify clients who would likely benefit from AHS services, and to match clients with types and levels of services appropriate for their health needs. The case management and case coordination system was developed to assure the continuity and appropriateness of care, to coordinate services among providers, and to terminate or modify the package of AHS services as necessary. The project developed and utilized a number of evaluation instruments for deciding those AHS services which were suitable for potential clients. These instruments, which were also used to collect research data, are discussed below (see "Research and Evaluation").

AHS client intake occurred at County Departments of Family and Children Services (DFACS), the major access points for state social services. These sites were selected for intake because DFACS workers were familiar with the target population's service needs.

An AHS caseworker based at a DFACS office administered the Client Assessment Interview (CAI) to the potential client and, whenever possible, a key person in the client's life, either a family member or friend. The CAI, data from the client's physician, and the caseworker's observation of the client's medical and social characteristics were all considered at a team conference involving a project-employed nurse, social worker, and caseworker. Of every four clients determined to be appropriate for alternative services, three were randomly assigned to the AHS experimental group and the fourth to a control group. Experimental group clients were referred to the appropriate service provider(s), who assessed them, determined the availability of service openings, and decided whether to offer the recommended services. Both experimental and control group clients remained eligible for any regular Medicaid, Title III, or Title XX services available in the target area.

During the period that services were provided, the AHS assessment team served as case manager, and the client's principal provider became case coordinator. As the case manager, the assessment team monitored client progress by reviewing and authorizing changes in categories of AHS services provided to a client. The case coordinator developed, updated (every 60 days) and shared the client's case plan with all agencies involved with the client's care. In addition, the case coordinator was responsible for day-to-day activities and problems relating to the client, including emergency placement.

Funding and Financing Mechanism

Sources. Funding for the AHS demonstration was provided through Section 1115(b) of the Social Security Act. During the demonstration, the project's administration and research activities were supported by nearly 100% Federal funding (5% state match was required during most years). Title XIX (Medicaid) funds were the primary source of Federal support for administration and research. Funding for project services (e.g., ALS, ADR, and HDS) was through the regular Medicaid program (approximately 67% Federal and 33% State). In addition, several caseworker positions were provided by Title XIX and the project, for a short period, used staff made available through the CETA program. Waivers granted to the project were as follows:

- *Waiver of statewideness.* This waiver enabled the State to limit the project to two of the State's ten regions.
- *Waiver of duration, amount, and scope of services.* This waiver allowed the project to offer nonstandard services under the demonstration and allowed project benefit services and program costs to be subject to the usual Medicaid Federal financial participation.
- *Waiver of eligibility standard (Title XIX).* This waiver permitted specified participants to remain in the project when they would have otherwise become ineligible themselves or made their spouses ineligible for Medicaid. For example, the waiver assured that those individuals who were eligible solely because

of their being in a nursing home and having income less than 300% of the SSI payment would remain Medicaid eligible when they participated in project alternative services.

Reimbursement method. All AHS providers were reimbursed for actual units of client service delivered, based on the cost to the provider for rendering the service. The AHS billing system provided for the processing of all AHS claims through the State of Georgia's Medicaid Management Information System (MMIS).

Services included in costs. All Medicaid and Medicare services were included in total direct service analyses. Separate analyses were conducted for estimating screening, assessment, and case management costs.

Cost containment approaches. Cost containment approaches to minimize the use of Medicaid funds included:

- Maximum Units of Service Guidelines which related service needs to costs were developed to help identify clients who required more intensive care than could be provided by the project in a cost-effective manner; e.g., costs for alternative health services would be higher than for nursing home care.
- A system of utilization review for community-based services was carried out by an independent review organization to assure that the amount, duration, scope and quality of services provided to AHS clients were appropriate.
- Audits of service providers were conducted to determine actual costs of services.

RESEARCH AND EVALUATION

Research Design and Data Collection

AHS was one of the first community-based demonstration projects, funded either under Section 222 Medicare waivers or Section 1115 Medicaid waivers, to utilize an experimental research design which employed random assignment of individuals to experimental and control groups. As described below, randomization occurred *after* a client was screened and determined to be appropriate for project services.

Data on client health and functional status, demographics, social supports, and other characteristics were obtained from the CAI administered prior to project enrollment. Follow-up interviews conducted at semi-annual intervals following enrollment provided the measure of relative changes. Measures on the CAI and follow-up interviews included mental status (Pfeiffer, 1975), morale (Lawton, 1975), walking independence and mobility (Katz, Ford, Downs, Adams, & Rusby, 1973), Activities of Daily Living (Katz, Downs, Cash, & Grotz, 1970), and Instrumental Activities of Daily Living (Lawton & Brody, 1969).

Cost and utilization data on health and related services were derived from AHS claims and other Medicaid billing records, and from Medicare and Title XX service records. All Medicaid and Medicare claim information for both AHS experimental and control group clients was retrieved from Georgia's Medicaid Management Information System (MMIS). Extensive processing of these claims was undertaken in order to prepare the data for the analyses.

Data collection began in late 1976 and continued through June 1980. Clients in both the experimental and control groups were tracked from the date of enrollment through the end of the demonstration period or until the client's death. Individual client data were transformed into 30-day intervals (months) or quarters (three 30-day intervals) from the client's team conference (enrollment date).

Most of the findings below are based on comparisons between the 444 experimental and 135 control group members in the "24-month sample." A full account of the project's research design, findings and recommendations can be found in the project's final report (Skellie, Favor, Tudor, & Strauss, 1982). In general, the project's research design allowed for the comparison of a system of community-based long term care with existing services available to individuals who were eligible for Medicaid-reimbursed nursing home care.

Findings

Project service utilization.

- About 80% of experimental group clients utilized an equivalent of at least two weeks of AHS project services during their first year of enrollment.
- The largest proportion (63%) of utilizers used home-delivered services (HDS); the lowest proportion (9%) used alternative

living services (ALS) alone or in conjunction with other services; 14% used a combination of adult day rehabilitation and home-delivered services.

- In general, clients living in facilities other than a private residence and clients who were never married were more likely to use ALS. Clients who were more independent in mobility and who received no outside supports were more likely to use ADR. Clients who were older, lived alone or with a spouse, had a diagnosis of heart disease, had been receiving support from caregivers, and did not go outside were more likely to use HDS.

Nursing home utilization and substitution.

- During the first two years following enrollment, only 22% of the control group and 21% of the experimental group were admitted to a nursing home. This is likely to be attributable to the voluntary nature of project participation and the fact that the target population included individuals considered to be ''at risk'' of nursing home admission but who had not necessarily applied for nursing home admission.
- For the experimental group as a whole, it appears that AHS services generally constituted additional Medicaid-reimbursed services rather than substitutes for nursing home care.
- However, there may have been some substitution of AHS services for nursing home care, particularly during the first six months after enrollment and for ALS recommendees.

Cost findings.

- Because AHS services in general tended to supplement rather than substitute for non-project services, average combined Medicaid-Medicare costs per client were found to be significantly higher for the experimental group than for the control group.
- But, because of the much lower average cost of AHS project services per quarter when compared to average nursing home costs per quarter, cost savings appear to be possible if project services can be substituted for nursing home services.
- Considerable variation in Medicaid and Medicare costs was found among clients recommended for each of the three categories of service (ALS, ADR, HDS).

- For both ADR and HDS recommendees, the experimental group's combined Medicaid and Medicare costs were significantly higher than such costs for control group clients (Figure 1).
- Further, a pattern of higher ALS control group costs after the third quarter of enrollment indicates a potential for cost savings beyond 24 months (Figure 2).

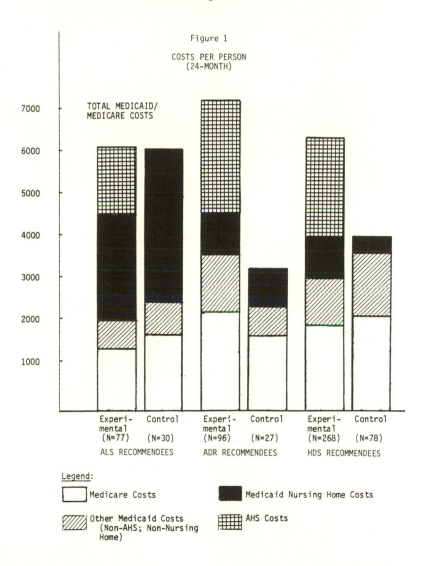

Figure 1

COSTS PER PERSON
(24-MONTH)

Figure 2

MEAN QUARTERLY MEDICAID-MEDICARE COSTS

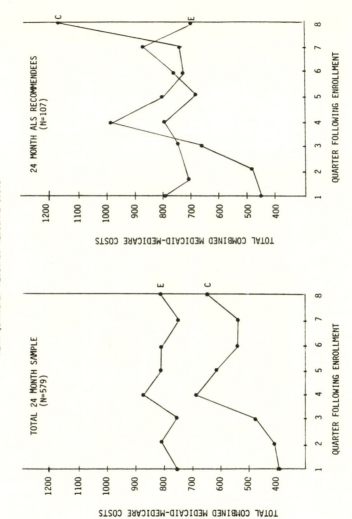

Note. Includes survivors and clients who died.

62

Effectiveness findings.

- Experimental group clients in general had a higher survival rate and lived longer on the average than control group clients. Six months after enrollment, 15% of control group clients had died as compared to 8% of experimental group clients; one year after enrollment, 22% of the control group and 14% of the experimental group had died. Both these differences are statistically significant at p < .05. At 24 months following enrollment, the difference in mortality rates, though not statistically significant, was 7% (Figure 3).
- The largest positive experimental effect in terms of survival was exhibited by clients recommended for HDS. The smallest differential in mortality between the experimental and control groups occurred for those clients recommended for ADR (Figure 3).
- No statistically significant differences between the total experimental and control groups were observed for any other outcome measures (ADL, IADL, Mental Status, Morale, Mobility, Walking), except for clients' perceptions of whether they were receiving enough help. Experimental group clients were more likely to indicate that they were receiving enough help than were control group clients.
- Experimental group clients recommended for ALS maintained a higher performance on ADL than did control group ALS recommendees.

LESSONS LEARNED

Of the lessons learned by the project, we have selected those we feel are most salient for long term care policy and most applicable to other community-based long term care programs. Formulated through five years of operational experience with the AHS project and from the evaluation findings summarized in the preceding pages, these recommendations relate to two areas:

- Client screening, placement, and case management; and
- Types of services provided, and monitoring and control of service providers.

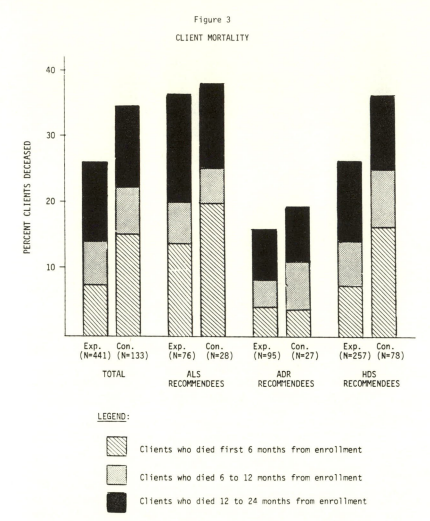

Figure 3

CLIENT MORTALITY

LEGEND:

Clients who died first 6 months from enrollment

Clients who died 6 to 12 months from enrollment

Clients who died 12 to 24 months from enrollment

Client Screening, Placement and Case Management

The most important lesson learned was the difficulty under a voluntary screening system of selecting individuals for whom community-based long term care would be most cost-effective. This selection problem, which requires the development of objective criteria, will be the subject of further discussion below (see "Discussion").

Another obstacle was a relatively low demand for project services. This low volume of clients screened and served resulted in higher administrative (screening, referral, and case management) and direct service costs. As a result of fewer referrals than expected, the administrative costs of enrolling clients into the project were estimated to be approximately three times higher than necessary. The low number of referrals had a particularly strong impact on the costs of services in freestanding adult day rehabilitation centers. Fixed minimum facility and staffing costs resulted in costs that were 25% or more higher than the optimum client census would have required.

A major recommendation based on the project's experience is that states implement programs of mandatory prescreening and assessment to determine appropriateness of community-based services for all Medicaid-eligible individuals who apply to nursing homes. This will allow a community-based program to concentrate on individuals who are most likely to enter a nursing home. In addition, actual applicants for nursing home care should provide a larger, more stable pool of referrals and should result in greater efficiency of screening, referral, case management and direct service provision than with a voluntary referral system.

Services Provided, Monitoring and Control

Another major difficulty experienced by the project was recruitment of providers. Providers were more likely to succeed in establishing a service if there were an existing parent agency; capability of covering cash flow and other resources; previous operating experience with a similar type of service; and sufficient, available staff. Financial incentives to cover start-up and growth costs are recommended if it is necessary to develop new providers. Fee-for-service reimbursement alone was a hardship for freestanding, independent new providers enrolled with the project.

The project kept close fiscal control over providers, including negotiating detailed line-item budgets in order to set service fees as close to actual cost as possible and minimize cost settlements. It is recommended that a system of prospective reimbursement be established once budgeted costs for providers begin to closely match actual costs.

Finally, it is strongly recommended that a utilization and quality review process be considered an essential element of any community-based alternatives program. The need to monitor the utilization and quality of services provided is as important in a non-institutional setting as in an institutional setting. The AHS Project utilization review procedures were developed from those used for institutional services. While the project's utilization review was a useful administrative tool, it was not based upon an integrated methodology or established criteria which could assure quality or appropriate utilization. Aside from the regulations governing certification requirements of Home Health Agencies for Medicare and Medicaid, no similar quality assurance programs are known to exist for community- or home-based long term care services. It is therefore recommended that research be undertaken to develop and test objective criteria and methodologies for the utilization and quality review of alternative services. An empirically based utilization review and quality assurance system should help maximize the probability that community-based services may be provided cost-effectively.

DISCUSSION: ISSUES IN POPULATION SELECTION

The primary objective of the AHS Project was to provide cost-effective community-based services to individuals certified as eligible for Medicaid-reimbursed nursing home care. The expectation was that project services would be at least as effective as institutional care and that the services would substitute for more costly institutional care. It was demonstrated that average Medicaid service costs per individual during the study period were lower than nursing home costs. However, it was also determined that the individuals served by the program generally would not have entered a nursing home, in the absence of project services. These findings suggest that nursing home eligibility alone is not a sufficient criterion for selection for community-based services.

The lower costs of project services compared to nursing home costs suggest that cost savings might be realized if the service target population is restricted to clients who were likely to substitute community-based services for nursing home care.

Since one of the major objectives of community-based alternatives to institutional care is to contain public expenditures for long term care services, the success of a program, in part, is dependent on its effectiveness in selecting a client population and in providing that population a combination of reasonably priced services that meet their varied health needs. Cost-effective care may be possible only if the service population is limited to clients who are likely to enter a nursing home and who are likely to utilize community-based alternatives as cost-effective substitute services. Identifying these individuals is necessary to the development of a community-based program.

Based on the AHS Project's experience, a number of points related to the issue of providing community-based long term care to the most appropriate population will be discussed. These include: (1) the need for standardized criteria for placement in either nursing home or community-based care; (2) the particular difficulty of objectively assessing the viability of social support networks and using this information for placement; (3) how mandatory prescreening of nursing home applicants can be a partial solution; and (4) suggestions for further research.

The Need for Standardized Criteria

Early reports from studies testing the cost-effectiveness of home health services suggested that considerable cost savings could be achieved by substituting home health for institutional services (Hammond, 1979). These conclusions were generally based on the judgment of health care professionals that in a certain percentage of cases community-based alternatives could have been substituted for nursing home care or hospitalization. Despite this optimism, selecting individuals for whom alternative care could substitute for nursing home care has proven to be difficult.

Research on long term care prediction models has focused on the development of algorithms and rating scales to predict the need for or predisposition to institutional care as well as the level of care required for community- or institutional-based settings (Grauer & Birnbom, 1975; Sherwood, Morris, Gutkin, & Wieners, 1977; Beckman, Noelker, & Debra, 1977; Orr, 1978; McAuley, Carnes, & Nutty, 1979; Greenberg & Ginn, 1979; Seidl, Applebaum, Austin, & Mahoney, 1980; Tudor, Favor, & Skellie, 1980). None of these prediction models, however, has been shown to select from among applicants to a community-based care program those who would enter a nursing home in the absence of alternative care. In three studies of community-based care which employed an experimental design, the community care was generally not found to have been provided to a nursing home bound group (Weissert, Wan, &

Livieratos, 1979; Seidl et al., 1980; Skellie et al., 1982). A major effort of the National Long-Term Care Demonstration ("Channeling") has been development of a screening instrument which is designed to select individuals more at risk of institutionalization (Carcagno & Kemper, 1981). Perhaps this effort will result in the objective criteria necessary for selecting those individuals most appropriate for community-based alternatives.

Consideration should also be given to revising the Medicaid nursing home admission criteria which certify as eligible a group of individuals who, for the most part, are not nursing home bound. Criteria for determining eligibility for Medicaid reimbursement for nursing home care are generally heavily weighted toward physical health status, seeking to determine if individuals are disabled enough to justify nursing home care. They do not consider either an individual's or family's motivation to keep the individual at home, nor generally information concerning the availability or viability of social supports. Objective assessment of the availability and viability of social supports is likely to be difficult (see next section). It is even more difficult to determine objectively factors that measure individuals' and families' intentions regarding entering a nursing home. A person may be disabled enough and have few enough supports to justify the need for the type of care provided in a long term care institution, yet have no intention of entering a nursing home. Because of the difference between eligibility for and intent to enter a nursing home, it is unlikely that revised nursing home admission criteria alone would be sufficient to ensure the selection of individuals who would substitute community care for nursing home care.

Objective Assessment of Social Supports

An important concern of community-based long term care programs is that these services may reduce the incentive of informal support networks to continue providing services to the elderly individual. These programs may not be cost-effective unless they supplement, rather than substitute for, informal services provided by an elderly individual's family or friends. Thus it is especially important that any placement decision take into consideration the viability of existing social support networks and determine what is needed either to maintain or develop these networks.

In the AHS Project, the best predictors of nursing home utilization were a request for Alternative Living Services and a report of applying for nursing home care (Tudor et al., 1980). Further, uncertainty of support by a key person was the best predictor of either nursing home utilization or death (Tudor, Favor, & Skellie, 1981). Probably the best predictor of entering a nursing home would be the direct question, "Do you plan to enter a nursing home?" Unfortunately, such a question could not be considered for an objective assessment, because it would be too easy for a respondent to provide the "correct" answer. Similarly, if availability of informal supports were used as a basis to deny eligibility for nursing home care, it seems likely that clients and families would tend to underestimate such support. Objective measures of the viability of social supports are needed, as well as standards for determining the level of support sufficient for a particular individual. Further understanding is needed of reasons why families or friends are unable to continue their support.

Only individuals with some informal supports can be provided home or day care at a public cost which is no more than the public cost of nursing home care. A question which must be answered, in order to determine the cost-effectiveness of alternatives to nursing home care, is "Are informal supports sufficient to keep an individual at home when some formal community-based care is added, yet insufficient by themselves to keep the person out of a nursing home?"

Mandatory Prescreening of Nursing Home Applicants

A voluntary screening system, based on the results of the AHS project and other studies, appears unlikely to provide a sufficient number of individuals at imminent risk of nursing home placement. Compared to nursing home applicants, volunteers for community-based services are likely to be less disabled and may constitute an add-on population rather than one for whom community-based services substitute for nursing home care.

A requirement that all applicants for Medicaid-reimbursed nursing home care be screened for appropriateness of community-based care offers a partial solution to the selection problem. Those applicants who are appropriate can be given a choice of community-based care. Mandatory prescreening of nursing home applicants ensures that both consumers and providers will be educated to the availability of long term care alternatives. Although it is still possible to apply for nursing home care in order to obtain alternative care, the proportion of "real" substitutions of alternatives for nursing home care should be considerably higher with prescreening of all Medicaid nursing home applicants.

Suggestions for Further Research

Further research to develop objective methods of assigning clients to services is strongly recommended. A three-step research strategy is suggested. First, develop a method to identify clients who are likely to enter a nursing home and who may be more likely to substitute community-based care for nursing home care. Second, develop selection criteria to identify the subgroup of nursing home bound elderly whose needs can be met by community-based services in a cost-effective manner. Last, develop criteria for determining which services are likely to be most effective for particular clients. Accomplishing the first two steps will require data from both nursing home applicants and volunteer applicants to a community-based long term care program.

Multivariate analyses of costs and effectiveness of the total package of AHS project services and of categories of services were generally inconclusive, but some further analysis of the project data by specific services (i.e., nursing, meals, etc.) within service categories has been undertaken. Findings from this analysis of eight specific service components indicated that home delivered meals, carefully targeted, may be cost-effective (Favor & Skellie, 1982). Among meal users who initially lived alone and needed a special diet, were dependent in ADL, or had impaired mental status, greater use of meals was associated with fewer nursing home days and lower Medicaid costs. The same approach may be applied to other service components, using different criteria for target groups. It is recommended that similar analysis be undertaken both of AHS and other demonstration project data, in order to identify characteristics of individuals for whom certain patterns of service may be cost-effective.

CONCLUSION

As a result of the AHS demonstration project, community-based long term care services have been incorporated into the Georgia Medicaid program. The present AHS program which is expanding statewide, incorporates a number of the recommendations made based on the project's experience. First, the State of Georgia will require mandatory prescreening for appropriateness of community-based care of all applicants for Medicaid-reimbursed nursing home care by 1985. Prospective reimbursement of providers has been adopted. Provider recruitment is now conducted by Area Agencies on Aging, through a bid process, using criteria developed by the project. The screening process has been simplified, and an automated management information system is being developed. Finally, multivariate analysis of the cost-effectiveness of specific project services has been conducted.

REFERENCES

Beckman, A. C., Noelker, L. S., & Debra, D. *Peer review: Overt and covert factors in the decision to institutionalize.* Paper presented at the annual meeting of the Gerontological Society, San Francisco, 1977.

Carcagno, G., & Kemper, P. *The evaluation design of the National Long Term Care Demonstration.* Paper presented at the annual meeting of the American Public Health Association, Los Angeles, November 1981.

Favor, F., & Skellie, F. A. *Cost-effectiveness of components of community-based long term care.* Paper presented at the annual meeting of the American Public Health Association, Montreal, November 1982.

Grauer, H., & Birnbom, F. A geriatric functional rating scale to determine the need for institutional care. *Journal of the American Geriatrics Society,* 1975, *23,* 472-476.

Greenberg, J., & Ginn, A. A multivariate analysis of the predictors of long term placement. *Home Health Care Services Quarterly,* 1979, *1,* 75-79.

Hammon, J. Home health care cost effectiveness: An overview of the literature. *Public Health Reports,* 1979, *94,* 305-311.

Katz, S., Downs, T. D., Cash, H., & Grotz, R. C. Progress in the development of the index of ADL. *The Gerontologist,* 1970, *10,* 20-30.

Katz, S., Ford, A. B., Downs, T. D., Adams, M., & Rusby, D. J. *Effects of continued care: A study of chronic illness in the home* (DHEW Publication No. (HSM) 73-3010). Washington, DC: U.S. Government Printing Office, 1973.

Lawton, M. P. The Philadelphia Geriatric Center morale scale: A revision. *Journal of Gerontology,* 1975, *30,* 85-89.

Lawton, M. P., & Brody, E. M. Assessment of older people: Self-maintaining and instrumental activities of daily living. *The Gerontologist,* 1969, *9,* 179-186.

McAuley, W. J., Carnes, C. C., & Nutty, C. L. *Multidisciplinary team decision regarding nursing home placement: A discriminant analysis.* Paper presented at the annual meeting of the Gerontological Society, Washington DC, 1979.

Orr, M. *Development of numerical standards for patient placement in New York State long term care facilities.* New York: Bureau of Research and Evaluation, New York State Office of Health Systems Management, 1978.

Pfeiffer, E. A short, portable mental status questionnaire for the assessment of organic brain deficits in elderly patients. *Journal of the American Geriatrics Society,* 1975, *23,* 433-441.

Seidl, F. W., Applebaum, R., Austin, C. D., & Mahoney, K. J. *Delivering in-home ser-*

vices to the aged and disabled: The Wisconsin Community Care Organization (Final evaluation report). Madison, Wisconsin: The University of Wisconsin, 1980.

Sherwood, S., Morris, J. N., Gutkin, C. E., & Wieners, C. N. Development of an easily applied screening instrument to identify elderly persons who would not be able to remain in the community without current informal supports. Boston: The Department of Social Gerontological Research, Hebrew Rehabilitation Center for Aged, 1977.

Skellie, F. A., Favor, F., Tudor, C., & Strauss, R. Alternative Health Services Final Report. Atlanta: Georgia Department of Medical Assistance, January 1982. (NTIS No. PB82-221128).

Tudor, C., Favor, F., & Skellie, F. A. Predictors of nursing home utilization in Georgia's Alternative Health Services Project: Preliminary findings. Paper presented at the Annual Meeting of the Gerontological Society of America, San Diego, CA, November 1980.

Tudor, C., Favor, F., & Skellie, F. A. Predictors of nursing home entry or death in Georgia's Alternative Health Services Project. Paper presented at the annual meeting of the American Public Health Association, Los Angeles, November 1981.

Weissert, W. G., Wan, T. T. H., & Livieratos, B. B. Effects and cost of day care and homemaker service for the chronically ill: A randomized experiment ((PHS) 79-3250). Hyattsville, MD: National Center for Health Services Research, August 1979.

Chapter 4

The South Carolina Community Long Term Care Project

Thomas E. Brown, MBA
R. Max Learner, PhD

OVERVIEW

The South Carolina Community Long Term Care Project (CLTC) is a Medicare and Medicaid research and demonstration project whose purpose is to provide information for planning state policies in long term care for elderly and disabled persons. The project's major objectives are to develop a system for assessment, care planning, case management, and reassessment; to test a number of expanded community services under Medicaid and Medicare; and to conduct research on topics in long term care. Among the issues to be studied are the effectiveness of service management and expanded Medicaid community services as long term care resources; hospital and nursing home utilization; and the cost-effectiveness of community-based long term care.

The CLTC project resulted from concerns that disabled South Carolinians had few resources for long term care, other than institutional care. Community-based services under Medicaid are very limited, and available only to the poorest Medicaid recipients. The State's two-tiered Medicaid system provides an incentive for institutionalization, in that persons with incomes between the Supplemental Security Income (SSI) level and 300% of the SSI level are eligible for Medicaid only as nursing home residents. In the CLTC project patients are given the option of receiving needed care at

Thomas E. Brown is Project Director and R. Max Learner is Director of Planning at South Carolina Community Long Term Care.

Questions may be directed to Thomas E. Brown, MBA, Project Director, South Carolina Community Long Term Care, 17-A Metro Drive, Spartanburg, SC 29303.

home or in an institution, and services can be varied along a continuum of care as their needs change.

The CLTC project began accepting clients in July 1980 under Medicaid 1115 waiver authority. During the first two years of implementation, over 2600 individuals were referred for admission; 1071 clients were active as of June 30, 1982. All of the expanded community-based services are in place. Beginning in 1983, the project will implement the Medicare portion of the experiment under Section 222 waiver authority, while continuing the Medicaid portion. The Medicare project will study the implications of changes in regulations that restrict Medicare payments for long term care services.

PROJECT ORIGIN AND OBJECTIVES

In 1978, the South Carolina General Assembly authorized funding for the CLTC project and formed the Long Term Care Policy Council for its coordination and overall policy direction. Council members include the Commissioners of the Departments of Social Services, Mental Health, Health and Environmental Control, and Mental Retardation; the Director of the Commission on Aging; and the Governor or his designee. The Council has responsibility for making recommendations to the Governor and the Legislature concerning necessary or desirable modifications within the State's long term care system. A Legislative Advisory Committee comprised of the Chairmen of six legislative committees affecting the elderly and long term care was also formed to support the CLTC program. The CLTC project's state level management and policy development structure provides a unique opportunity for transferring positive project findings to a statewide program.

The CLTC project grew out of earlier policy planning and research activities. In 1973, the South Carolina Commission on Aging contracted with the University of South Carolina to perform a statewide study of institutional services for the elderly. The study priorities included collecting fiscal and patient data from long term care institutions in the state; investigating possible alternatives that might permit deinstitutionalization or prevent early institutionalization; and developing recommendations regarding long term care services. Recommendations for expanded community-based services that would reduce the need for institutional services resulted. In

1977, the Task Force on Long Term Care examined the rising costs of institutional long term care under the Medicaid program and reached a similar conclusion.

Thus, in 1977, the Chairman of the South Carolina General Assembly's Study Committee on Aging initiated a Task Force to develop a model project on community-based services. The Task Force included representatives from various state agencies and other organizations involved in institutional care. After study of programs in other states with client assessment, case management, and community-based services, the Task Force produced plans for a demonstration project. In the spring of 1978, the General Assembly authorized funding for the CLTC project in a three-county area.

A small grant from the Appalachia Regional Commission supported the planning for the CLTC project during the 1978-1979 Fiscal Year. The initial project proposal for Section 1115 Medicaid and Section 222 Medicare waivers was submitted to the Health Care Financing Administration (HCFA) of the Department of Health and Human Services (HHS) in June 1979. The project received conditional approval of Section 1115 Medicaid waivers in November 1979 and final approval in July 1980. The Medicare 222 waiver program was approved in October 1982 and scheduled for implementation in April 1983.

The CLTC project is located administratively within the Department of Social Services, South Carolina's Medicaid agency, with the CLTC Project Director responsible to the Commissioner of the Department of Social Services. In the three-county demonstration area, the CLTC office is a separate, freestanding unit. Memoranda of agreement (MOA) have been developed with the local agency counterparts of Long Term Care Policy Council participants. These MOA identify the local line agency's and the CLTC project's area of responsibility, coordination and cooperation.

From July 1, 1979 to July 16, 1980, preoperational activities were accomplished to prepare for the experimental phase's implementation. For example, through a new mandatory pre-admission screening program for nursing home applicants seeking Medicaid benefits, needs assessments, level of care determinations and care plans were completed for 726 clients. Contracts for services also were developed; staff was recruited; the assessment instrument was tested; service management was implemented with existing community services; and the service management system was further developed.

PROJECT CHARACTERISTICS

The CLTC project is located in Spartanburg, Cherokee, and Union Counties which contain approximately 9% of the state's population (U.S. Bureau of the Census, 1981) and rural and urban areas typical of South Carolina. Spartanburg County, with the largest population of the three (201,553 in 1980) has a sizeable urban center, the city of Spartanburg (population of 43,968) and two other towns with populations of 2500 or more. Cherokee County, population 40,983, is mainly rural with one major town, Gaffney (population 13,453). Union County, population 30,751 is largely rural. Its largest town is the county seat, Union, with 10,523 persons (U.S. Bureau of Census, 1981).

Comparisons between the counties with regard to medical-service availability reflect a rural/urban division. Cherokee and Union Counties have been designated as medical manpower shortage areas, with the 1978 population to primary care physician ratio in these counties (3,863:1) almost twice as high as that for Spartanburg (2,058:1). Each county has an adequate number of hospital beds, although the ratio of population to hospital bed is much lower for Spartanburg (51:1) than either Union (193:1) or Cherokee (254:1). Long term institutional care is available in each county (occupancy rate: 99%), with seven nursing homes in Spartanburg and two each in Cherokee and Union.

Community services for the disabled elderly were available in each county: home health services, through the Department of Health and Upjohn Health Services; Medicaid, Title XX, and Food Stamps through the Department of Social Services; Title III services through the Commission on Aging; and a large voluntary home-delivered meals program serving Spartanburg County.

Population Served

CLTC project clients must be aged 18 or older, live in the project area, have functional dependencies in two areas of activities of daily living (or meet the level of care criteria for nursing home admission), and meet Medicaid eligibility requirements. The CLTC's mandatory preadmission screening policy provides a standard evaluation of a patient's need for a nursing home level of care and ensures that all who attempt to obtain Medicaid long term care services will access the CLTC project.

Of the 2604 individuals referred to the CLTC project between July 17, 1980 and June 30, 1982, 2236 received initial assessments and 1357 were accepted as project participants. The major reasons for client attrition were the decision not to participate, death, and Medicaid ineligibility. Demographic data describing project participants are presented in Table 1. The majority of participants,

Table 1

BASELINE CHARACTERISTICS BY GROUP

	Control Group (n=337)	Experimental Group (n=282)	Statistical Test
Age			
Mean age	74.87	73.23	t=1.48
Standard deviation	13.35	12.91	
n	333	277	
Race and Sex			X^2 =3.42
White female	58%	58%	
White male	21	21	
Black female	12	15	
Black male	9	6	
Marital Status			X^2 =1.60
Married	27	32	
Widowed/Divorced	64	59	
Never married	9	9	
Household Composition			X^2 =6.91
Lives alone	23	23	
Spouse	25	32	
Child	31	23	
Other	21	22	
Monthly Income			X^2 = .55
$ 0-99	6	5	
$100-199	15	17	
$200-299	51	50	
$300-399	19	20	
$400 and above	9	9	
Initial Medicaid Eligibility Status			X^2 = .21
Categorical	30	28	
Medical Assistance Only	70	72	
Initial Level of Care			X^2 =1.85
Skilled nursing care	64	60	
Intermediate care	36	40	

Note. Year 1 cohort, patients at SNF or ICF Initial Level of Care. Chi-square tests for homogeneity were made using frequency data; percentages were reported in the table for ease of interpretation.

82%, were at nursing home levels of care. Women represented 69% of the clients and the average age was 74 years.

Service Program

The CLTC has initiated service management for all experimental clients, expanded community services for experimental clients who chose to remain at home, reassessed control clients, developed new services and negotiated agreements with existing service agencies. Community advisory committees in each county and ongoing communication between project staff and the participating agencies were used to enlist service provider and community cooperation.

Assessment. Nurses and social workers on the project staff perform all initial assessments which cover physical and mental health status, demographic characteristics, functional abilities, social supports, and service needs. Following the initial assessment, clients who meet project admission criteria are randomly assigned to the control or experimental group. Controls who wish to remain in the community are referred to the existing system of community agencies for services and case management. Reassessments are performed at 90 days after initial assessment, 180 days, one year, and six month intervals thereafter for both groups.

Service management. Besides assessment, experimental participants received ongoing service management by the CLTC project staff. The nurse-social worker service management team provides the necessary expertise for helping clients meet their medical and social needs. The team is responsible for certifying level of care, preparing care plans, authorizing and coordinating expanded services, monitoring the implementation of care plans, and performing scheduled reassessments. Service managers remain available as contact persons and resources, able to adapt the plan of care whenever changes in the patients' condition or family circumstances occur. This flexibility, along with periodic reassessment and reevaluation of care plans, means that experimental patients can move quickly into the services they need at a particular point in time and receive an appropriate level of care.

Available services. The CLTC project's expanded community-based services include: personal care; medical day care; home delivered meals; medical social services; physical, speech and occupational therapy; respite care; and expanded Medicaid eligibility for clients with incomes up to 300% of the SSI.

Personal care, the most heavily used service by community-based experimental clients at a nursing home level of care, includes support for activities of daily living (i.e., bathing, personal grooming, hygiene, meal planning and preparation, transfer, ambulation); housekeeping (i.e., light cleaning, laundry, shopping, home safety); and medical monitoring of the client.

Medical day care services include checking vital signs, monitoring medication, providing instruction in self-care, coordinating treatment plans with the client's physician, medical social services, physical therapy, training in activities of daily living, planned therapeutic activities, occupational therapy, one meal and a snack daily, supervision of personal care, and transportation to and from the center.

Existing home-delivered meal programs serve most of the meals. In one county (Cherokee), a Medicaid-sponsored contract for therapeutic and regular home-delivered meals supplement these ongoing programs.

Respite care, temporary nursing home placement for up to 14 days per year, is intended to relieve primary caregivers from patient care. Respite contracts have been implemented with nursing homes in the area.

Medical social services and expanded home health services (physiotherapy, occupational therapy, and speech therapy) are not new in the community but prior to their coverage as waivered services were not fully available to community-based long term care patients. Expanded eligibility for regular Medicaid benefits enables inclusion of clients who would have been eligible for Medical Assistance Only (MAO) only if in a nursing home. This group, which includes over 50% of the experimentals, are able to receive regular community-based Medicaid services, such as physician visits, drugs, outpatient therapies, etc. A monthly, sliding scale copayment is charged to MAO-type experimentals who wish these regular Medicaid services.

Funding and Financing Mechanism

The CLTC project is being implemented under the authority of Medicaid and Medicare waivers. Sources of funding include Federal Medicaid, Medicare, State and the Appalachia Regional Commission.

The Medicaid and Medicare waivers include:

- Waiver of statewideness (Medicaid).
- Waiver of amount, duration, and scope of services (Medicaid and Medicare).
- Waiver of coverage for the cost of services not otherwise subject to Federal financial participation (Medicaid).
- Waiver of specific home health services requirements (Medicare).
- Waiver of specific skilled nursing home coverage requirements (Medicare).
- Waiver to permit coverage of expanded services including personal care, medical day care and other services (Medicare).

CLTC providers are reimbursed for the provision of waivered services by one of two methods: (1) interim rate, with a final settlement after the close of the contract, and (2) prospective rate.

Three operational policies being implemented in the CLTC model will be closely examined as potential cost containment measures. The mandatory preadmission screening/assessment for persons applying for Medicaid nursing home benefits is one. The second involves separating level of care decisions (i.e., skilled, intermediate or less than intermediate level of care) from those regarding best and most desirable location of care. Both the mandatory preadmission screening program and this service planning approach are directed toward intercepting individuals prior to their entering a nursing home and providing realistic choices about where their care will occur. The third CLTC policy requires the pricing out of community care plans. The CLTC service manager may authorize the use of waivered services up to 75% of the cost for the client if he were admitted to a long term care facility for a 90-day period. The cost of community services thus is related to the prevailing costs of institutional care and based on the client's level of care. That is, for clients at a skilled level of care, more CLTC services may be authorized than for clients at intermediate or less than intermediate levels of care.

RESEARCH AND EVALUATION

Research Design

The CLTC project is a longitudinal experiment with clients randomly assigned to control and experimental groups following their initial assessments and prior to Medicaid eligibility determination

(50% to each group). The project's experimental design permits comparisons of clients who receive service management and other new services with those served within the regular Medicaid system. The principal area of investigation is the CLTC program's impact on client outcomes and service utilization. To examine the cost and effectiveness of community-based services in meeting the needs of health impaired and disabled persons, experimental and control group outcomes will be compared, controlling for initial level of care, initial location of care, and baseline client characteristics as required.

Special studies also are being conducted using project data and other data bases to examine long term care policy issues and to provide a basis for program and policy decisions. Major issues include: the long term care population's characteristics; service utilization patterns; system-level impacts of the CLTC project on Medicaid service utilization and costs; potential impact of statewide implementation of the CLTC program on Medicaid expenditures and nursing home and community services utilization; the effects of modifying eligibility criteria (i.e., expanded eligibility for MAO-type patients, eligibility for less than ICF patients) on Medicaid expenditures; the implications of an integrated Medicare/Medicaid linkage for policy and programs; control of long term care costs; and the effects of community-based long term care on family and social supports.

Initial research activities have focused on nursing home utilization and health status of project clients admitted between July 1980 and June 1981, the first operational year. Data were available for up to 12 months of each client's participation, from the date of initial assessment until termination, death, or the end of one year. Four waves of client assessment data were obtained for survivors of the period.

Findings

The participant groups' demographic characteristics showed no significant differences with regard to age, race, sex, marital status, income, initial level of care, or initial Medicaid eligibility status (see Table 1). Studies of nursing home use and health status change were made, based on data from the subgroup of patients who met medical criteria for nursing home admission (SNF or ICF level of care) at the time of initial assessment. Complete data were available for 282 experimental and 337 control clients.

At initial assessment, the project groups were compared on indices of mental functioning, mobility and ability to perform activities of daily living and instrumental activities. Table 2 shows the results of these comparisons.

A version of Kahn's Mental Status Questionnaire (MSQ), a ten-item scale measuring orientation to place and time, was used as the mental status index. At initial assessment, there was no significant difference between the groups' mean MSQ scores for respondents at

Table 2

BASELINE COMPARISONS OF GROUPS ON FUNCTIONAL IMPAIRMENT MEASURES [a]
ACCORDING TO INITIAL LEVEL OF CARE

| Measure | Initial Level of Care | | | | | |
| | Skilled Nursing | | | Intermediate Care | | |
	Control (n=214)	Exper. (n=164)	T	Control (n=123)	Exper. (n=118)	T
Mental Status Questionnaire						
Mean Score	3.63 (n=150)	3.54 (n=123)	.21	3.68 (n=106)	3.15 (n=111)	1.22
Mobility Index						
Mean Score	4.17 (n=214)	4.19 (n=164)	-.10	2.74 (n=123)	2.00 (n=118)	2.69**
Activities of Daily Living						
Mean Score	8.25 (n=214)	8.14 (n=164)	.28	6.17 (n=123)	4.86 (n=116)	2.98**
Instrumental Activities of Daily Living						
Mean Score	9.69 (n=210)	9.04 (n=162)	.07	9.67 (n=123)	8.82 (n=118)	2.19*

[a] The higher the score, the higher the level of impairment.

*$p \leq .05$
**$p \leq .01$

either SNF or ICF level of care. Possible scores ranged from 0 errors (no impairment) to 10 errors. Many clients (approximately 26% of controls and 20% of experimentals) were unable to respond to the MSQ due to the severity of their illness or mental impairment.

Experimental clients at SNF level were comparable with SNF controls in mobility and in the performance of activities of daily living (ADL) and of instrumental activities of daily living (IADL). The mobility index was composed of items on ambulation, transfer and wheelchair use and ranged from 0 (no impairment) to 6 (complete dependence on others). The ADL scale was comprised of six items on bathing, dressing, eating, toileting, transfer, and continence. The IADL scale included six items on meal preparation, housekeeping, handling finances, shopping, taking medication and telephone use. Scores on the ADL and IADL scales ranged from 0 (no or minimal impairment) to 12 (severe impairment in all activities).

Although all participants were disabled to the extent that they were medically eligible for admission to ICF facilities, experimental ICF participants as a group were less functionally impaired than controls. ICF controls had significantly higher mobility, ADL, and IADL scores at initial assessment. These differences appear to be an artifact of sample selection and greater subject attrition within the ICF control group during the Medicaid eligibility process, due to a lack of incentives for continued participation.

Mortality and change in level of care. Since the population under study included many terminally ill patients, mortality was a major factor over the course of the client year (Table 3). Mortality and change in level of care over time were examined according to initial level of care. As shown in Table 3, among both levels of patients, the experimental and control groups showed similar patterns of change.

At the SNF level, approximately 40% of control patients and 34% of experimentals died during the 12 months following initial assessments. Death rates were lower among ICF level patients: 17% of controls and 18% of experimentals died during the one-year interval.

Comparisons between the groups based on initial level of care showed no significant differences in the distribution of level of care at any point in time.

Nursing home admissions. To measure use of nursing home resources, the participant groups were compared on the proportion of clients who entered nursing homes and the proportion of days spent

Table 3

SUBJECT MORTALITY AND LEVEL OF CARE AT ASSESSMENT INTERVALS

	Initial Assessment	90-Day Assessment	180-Day Assessment	365-Day Assessment
SNF Controls (n=214)				
SNF	100%	55%	41%	23%
ICF		16	20	20
Less than ICF		4	4	9
Dead		21	29	40
Terminated/Status Unknown		5	7	8
SNF Experimentals (n=164)				
SNF	100%	54%	37%	26%
ICF		21	22	22
Less than ICF		5	9	9
Dead		14	24	34
Terminated/Status Unknown		5	7	9
ICF Controls (n=123)				
SNF	100%	15%	20%	18%
ICF		62	51	38
Less than ICF		10	11	15
Dead		6	8	17
Terminated/Status Unknown		6	11	13
ICF Experimentals (n=118)				
SNF	100%	17%	13%	19%
ICF		67	52	40
Less than ICF		13	19	19
Dead		3	14	18
Terminated/Status Unknown		2	3	5

in nursing homes. Participation days included the number of days from initial assessment until termination, death or the end of the client's first year, thus taking subject mortality into account. Community days included days spent in hospitals, boarding homes, and at home.

The groups were compared on the proportions of clients who were admitted to nursing homes during the one-year period. Among all 282 experimental clients, 43% entered a nursing home at some time during the first year following initial assessment. The comparable figure for the 337 control clients was 57%. A test for equality of proportions indicated that the difference was significant ($Z = 3.5, p \leq .001$).

Further comparisons were made according to initial level of care to control for the differences in the composition of the groups. Although a greater percentage of controls at SNF level were admitted, the difference was not statistically significant. Among ICF level patients, however, a significantly greater proportion of control clients entered nursing homes: 56% compared with 34% of experimentals ($Z = 3.4, p \leq .001$). The findings showed that similar proportions of control clients at SNF and ICF levels entered nursing homes. Among experimental clients, a greater proportion of SNF patients used nursing home care than did persons at ICF level. This result suggests that the experimental program had a greater impact on nursing home admission among ICF level patients.

The comparisons of nursing home days used by participants showed that control clients at each level of care received significantly more days of nursing home care (see Table 4). Overall, 44% of the controls' participation days were spent in nursing homes, compared with 27% for experimental patients. The difference was particularly striking among patients at an ICF level of care. For ICF controls, 42% of the participation days were in nursing homes while only 20% of the ICF experimental-client days were spent in nursing homes.

Change in functional health status. Because a substantial proportion of clients died or terminated their participation, comparisons of change in functional health status were based on a subset of 185 control clients and 174 experimental clients who participated over the entire year. No significant differences were found with regard to race and sex, marital status, income level, or initial level of care although control participants were significantly older on the average ($t = 2.76, p \leq .01$).

Comparisons on ADL scores according to initial level of care were made at baseline and at 90-, 180-, and 365-day assessment intervals. Among participants initially at a SNF level of care, there were no significant differences on mental status, mobility, activities of daily living or instrumental activities of daily living measures at baseline or subsequent assessments. Among patients initially classified at ICF level, the control group was significantly more impaired on the ADL measure at baseline, with a mean of 6.14 compared to 5.04 for experimental ICF patients. However, the differences at subsequent assessments were not significant. The baseline dif-

Table 4

CHI-SQUARE COMPARISONS OF NURSING HOME DAYS
BY PARTICIPANT GROUP AND INITIAL LEVEL OF CARE

	Participant Days		
	Nursing Home	Community	Total
Participant Group			
Control (n=337)	41,572 (44%)	53,683 (56%)	95,255 (100%)
Experimental (n=282)	22,178 (27%)	60,464 (73%)	82,642 (100%)
X^2 =5435.***			
Skilled Nursing Patients			
Control (n=204)	24,868 (45%)	30,912 (55%)	55,780 (100%)
Experimental (n=164)	14,423 (32%)	30,073 (68%)	44,496 (100%)
X^2 =1538.***			
Intermediate Care Patients			
Control (n=123)	16,704 (42%)	22,771 (58%)	39,475 (100%)
Experimental (n=118)	7,745 (20%)	30,391 (80%)	38,136 (100%)
X^2 =4355.***			

***$p \leq .001$

ferences were taken into account in other analyses through use of initial ADL scores as a covariate.

An analysis of covariance was conducted to evaluate the main and interaction effects of group, initial level of care, and locus at one year (community versus nursing home) on one-year ADL scores, adjusted for initial ADL scores. Initial ADL accounted for most of the variance explained by the model (adjusted R^2 = .38). The findings indicated that, after adjusting for the effects of initial ADL score, nursing home patients were significantly more impaired than community-based patients on one-year ADL scores and no significant differences existed between the participant groups or between initial levels of care. Consequently, there was no evidence that the experimental intervention was more or less effective than the existing system experienced by the control group in improving patient functioning. Although the three-way interaction effect was not significant, experimental SNF patients in the community at one year improved by 2.28 points on the ADL measure from an initial mean of 7.23 to 4.95 at one year, while control SNF patients in the community improved from 5.86 to 5.12 in the group mean. No comparable finding was obtained among ICF patients.

Conclusion

Preliminary findings in the CLTC study indicate that the experimental intervention is successful in providing community-based care for long term care patients without adverse effects on patients' health. The comparisons between control and experimental participants revealed no important differences in mortality rates, patterns of change in level of care, or in ADL scores over a one-year interval. In both groups, clients who survived the year showed a small degree of improvement in ADL functioning. However, experimental clients used less nursing home care. In both the experimental and control groups, clients who remained in the community were characterized by lower levels of functional impairment than clients who used nursing home care. Among patients initially at nursing home levels of care, a greater proportion of experimental patients remained in the community; and for those clients who were admitted to nursing homes, experimental patients used less patient days of nursing home care.

Additional analyses are planned with larger samples over longer periods of time in order to examine more thoroughly the effects of community-based long term care on clients' health status. Further study is needed to specify the characteristics of patients for whom community services are most effective and those for whom nursing home services are most effective in promoting or maintaining health.

DISCUSSION: COORDINATING MEDICAID AND MEDICARE BENEFITS

For users, the Medicare and Medicaid programs present a maze of eligibility criteria, differences in reimbursable services, duplication of some services, and gaps in coverage for others. Regulations and needs are often in conflict, and clients are compelled to accept services they do not need, while going without appropriate alternatives. The effectiveness of both programs is reduced by the entanglement of eligibility criteria and service coverage. All of these inadequacies and problems clearly document the need for a coordination of acute and skilled care benefits of Medicare with those of Medicaid.

By project admission criteria, all of the CLTC project participants are eligible for Medicaid. A large proportion of the project's participants are also eligible for Medicare benefits. In many cases, the requirements of one program, i.e., either Medicare or Medicaid, cause unnecessary and/or increased costs in the other program. The CLTC project proposes to address several of these issues through implementation of both Medicaid (1115) waivers and Medicare (222) waivers during FY83-84. CLTC participants will continue to require either skilled or intermediate level long term care services as an admission criterion. Also, potential participants will continue to be identified through the state's mandatory preadmission screening program for Medicaid sponsored nursing home care. Although the primary focus of the research will remain on Medicaid costs, particular attention will be paid to the process by which clients become Medicaid sponsored nursing home patients.

A system for early identification of long term care needs through referrals by hospital personnel and community service agencies will be implemented. Upon referral, the project staff will perform a comprehensive assessment and evaluation, determine the level of care, develop a care plan if community placement is appropriate, and provide case management for experimental patients. Through this process, many individuals will be able to choose between community and nursing home placement as a setting for receiving their long term care services. Availability of coordinated service benefits from the two programs will improve services to the eligible population and, at the same time, improve the effectiveness of the two programs and conserve resources.

Under current policies, individuals who are hospitalized may be transferred to a nursing home with Medicare benefits if they are at skilled nursing level of care and if they are receiving follow-up care in the nursing home for the condition for which they were hospitalized. CLTC project experience to date has been that within a very short period of time, most individuals convert from Medicare to Medicaid. At that point, the State's preadmission screening program is accessed to determine the medical necessity for nursing home care. The project has found that in only a few cases will the patient choose community services as an option. The choice to continue institutional care is based primarily on the loss of the social support system which may have been present prior to institutionalization and, in some cases, the loss of a residence to which the patient could return. The CLTC project asserts that through the availability of both Medicare and Medicaid community services and the opportunity for early detection as outlined above, many individuals who presently choose nursing home care reimbursed through Medicare will choose to receive Medicare-funded community-based services.

Medicare was designed as a health insurance program to help disabled persons and patients aged 65 and older to defray costs of acute hospital care and the cost of short periods of convalescence in skilled care facilities. However, the lack of Medicare coverage for convalescence and follow-up care has led to inappropriate use of expensive hospital services. For many patients, this may lead to depletion of private resources and conversion to Medicaid. The magnitude of this problem in 1979 in the three-county CLTC project area was significant. Data from the South Carolina Medical Care Foundation (PSRO) indicated that approximately one-third of the hospital days for Medicare/Medicaid patients were alternate care days, i.e., days beyond acute care. Questions regarding the availability of skilled nursing beds for Medicare patients and the relative lack of Medicare-funded, community service options should be explored as possible causes for this problem.

Therefore, the CLTC project proposes to extend or expand Medicare coverage in order to provide community-based medical services which will reduce the need for dependency on acute hospital care. The development of community service options funded by Medicare, as well as the use of nursing home services for this target group will be evaluated through the CLTC project's data system and evaluation design. Outcome measures such as the use of community services, the use of nursing home services, and the appropriate use of hospital services will be available to answer this key policy question. The ability to access Medicare funded community-based long term care services will also affect Medicare to Medicaid conversion in nursing homes.

Chapter 5

The New York City Home Care Project: A Demonstration in Coordination of Health and Social Services

Roberta S. Brill, MSAM
Amy Horowitz, DSW

OVERVIEW

The New York City Department for the Aging's Home Care Project (HCP) is a research and demonstration program that provides home care and other needed maintenance level services to homebound, chronically ill elderly in four selected areas of New York City.

Unlike many other states where long term home care services are not available to any group within the population, New York State has covered personal care services as part of its Medicaid program since 1973. New York City in particular has made extensive use of this benefit, serving some 35,000 Medicaid recipients requiring maintenance level care at a cost of $347 million in 1981 (Raphael, 1982). Complementing this program is a large system of predominantly short-term home health care provided by certified home health agencies, including visiting nurse agencies and hospital-based departments. The certified agencies, while providing some long term services to Medicaid recipients, direct most of their services to

Roberta S. Brill is Project Director and Amy Horowitz is Senior Research Associate at the New York City Home Care Project.

This project is funded by the U.S. Health Care Financing Administration (Grant No. 95-P-97492/03) and the Administration on Aging (Grant No. 90-AM-2187/03).

The authors would like to acknowledge the contribution of John E. Dono, MA, Research Associate for the Project, to the analysis and interpretation of the data presented within this paper.

Questions may be directed to Roberta S. Brill, Project Director of the New York City Home Care Project, NYC Department for the Aging, 280 Broadway, New York, NY 10007.

Medicare patients with short-term intermittent skilled nursing or rehabilitative needs. For less impaired clients, the New York City Department for the Aging uses Older Americans Act funds to provide limited amounts of housekeeper or homemaker service to approximately 2,000 persons annually. The target population has been those elderly living on incomes marginally above Medicaid.

The HCP is jointly funded by the U.S. Health Care Financing Administration (HCFA) and the Administration on Aging (AoA). It is testing a community-based approach to the delivery of health and social services to homebound, chronically disabled elderly who are unable to obtain in-home services under present Medicare regulations. The program's overall aim is to enable participants to maintain a satisfactory existence at home and to prevent or defer unnecessary institutionalization. As of March 1983, the HCP had served 676 clients since its implementation in December 1980.

PROJECT ORIGIN AND OBJECTIVES

During 1979, the year in which the HCP proposal was developed, the Health Systems Agency of New York calculated that 102,400 people received publicly funded in-home services in New York City (HSA, 1977): 21,600 receiving personal care services on a long term basis and 57,500 receiving primarily short-term care through the certified home health agencies. An additional 17,900 clients received housekeeper and homemaker services through Medicaid, and 5,400 clients received Title 111B home care services through the New York City Department for the Aging.

Despite the size of the population served, the vast majority of the City's elderly are not eligible, by virtue of income, for publicly assisted home care benefits. Approximately 50% of the 951,732 New York City residents over 65 had incomes between $4,000 and $10,000, making them "near poor" and yet ineligible for Medicaid. Several surveys and studies in the City during the early to mid-1970s pointed to the need for coordination of existing services as well as extended in-home care for the "near poor" Medicare beneficiary (e.g., Cantor et al., 1970; Engler, 1978; HSA, 1977).

In 1978, as a first step to addressing the dual problem of limited and fragmented service, Mayor Edward I. Koch appointed a Task Force on Medical Home Health Care for the Elderly, composed of top level City officials representing health and social services. The

Task Force worked with the New York City Department for the Aging to develop a HCP grant application around the concept of coordinated service delivery through intersystem coordination and the provision of additional home care services. Intersystem coordination would take place at two levels: (1) at the City-wide level where the Department for the Aging, a federally-designated Area Agency on Aging and part of the municipal government, would take a lead role in more effectively coordinating service delivery to the City's elderly; and (2) at the community level where service coordination on behalf of individual clients would take place.

In September 1979 the New York City Department for the Aging was funded by the Administration on Aging to plan and implement the project design, establish HCP policies, oversee operations, collect the data and conduct an evaluation for the City's government. Three months later a grant was awarded by the Health Care Financing Administration. The start-up period extended through much of 1980. Community agencies were screened in order to select the four service delivery sites, the HCP design was finalized and Medicare waivers were approved by the Health Care Financing Administration.

Specific site selection criteria included: (1) demographic considerations, such as density of "marginal income" persons entitled to Medicare but not eligible for Medicaid within the catchment area; (2) borough considerations in order to give the HCP maximum visibility and to ensure that one site served a predominantly minority population; (3) organizational considerations, such as service capability and past performance, cooperation with other resources in the community, fiscal and accounting capability, and a commitment of top agency administration to the HCP; and (4) ability and willingness of a site to support the research needs.

Two health agencies and two social service agencies were selected, allowing the opportunity to document any differential experiences in delivering and coordinating services to a homebound population. These agencies, though established, were new to the provision of long term home health care services. They were: (1) the Community Agency for Senior Citizens (CASC) of the Community Service of N.Y., a social service agency serving Staten Island; (2) Comprehensive Family Care Center (CFCC) of the Albert Einstein College of Medicine, a freestanding ambulatory health care center serving parts of the Bronx; (3) the Jamaica Service Program for Older Adults (JSPOA), a social service agency serving Jamaica,

Queens; and (4) the Sunset Park Family Health Center (or FHC) of the Lutheran Medical Center, a hospital-based ambulatory health care facility serving parts of Brooklyn.

The HCP's objectives were to:

- Develop a cost effective model of coordinated service delivery for a homebound elderly population which can be incorporated within the City or other communities;
- Demonstrate a process of local and city-wide coordination of existing health care and social service resources on behalf of the homebound elderly to achieve maximum utilization of resources;
- Develop a documented knowledge base regarding the services needed by a homebound, chronically ill, elderly population as these relate to their disability levels; the cost of delivering such care; and the effects of this care, comparing the HCP population with a group not receiving HCP services.

PROJECT CHARACTERISTICS

Population Served

Each of the sites served a census of 100 clients in its catchment area. Beginning in December 1980 (at the first site) and between January and June 1981 (at the remaining three), clients meeting the following eligibility criteria were admitted: (1) over 65 years of age; (2) Medicare Part B eligible; (3) homebound to the extent that they were unable to go outside without assistance and/or needed help in carrying out activities of daily living; and (4) residing within the catchment area.

As discussed below in the Research and Evaluation section, longitudinal data are being collected from a research sample of 504 HCP clients and 200 matched comparisons.[1] The major demographic characteristics of both the client and the comparison groups are presented in Table 1. The client population is approximately two-thirds female (69%); primarily White (78%); over 75 years of age (68%);

---

[1]While sites continued to admit and collect data on new clients after March 1982 to fill their caseloads to the maximum of 100, these clients were not included in the data base since they could not be followed for a minimum of one year.

and of marginal income (66% with household incomes under $700 per month). Few differences emerge between the client and comparison groups with the exception of race, which reflects the intentional selection of one site serving primarily minority clients (Jamaica Service Program for Older Adult's caseload is 72% Black).

As shown in Table 1, almost half (45%) the client population were married; two-thirds (64%) lived with others, primarily family members; 71% had at least one child; and of those with children

Table 1

BASELINE CLIENT CHARACTERISTICS BY GROUP

	Clients	Comparison
Age		
65-74	32%	28%
75-84	44	48
85+	24	25
(n)	(504)	(200)
Mean	78.3	79.1
Sex		
Male	31	32
Female	69	68
(n)	(504)	(200)
Race		
White	78	87
Black	19	10
Other	3	4
(n)	(504)	(200)
Marital Status		
Married	45	48
Living Situation		
Alone	36	41
With Others	64	59
Social Network		
Has at least one living child	71	68
Has at least one close relative	88	89
Has at least one close friend	59	55
Frequency of Contact with Children		
At least 5 days per week or lives with child	64	69
At least weekly	25	24
Less than weekly	12	7
Monthly Income		
Under $500	38	36
$500 - $699	29	27
$700+	34	37
(n)	(493)	(192)

64% either lived with a child or were in contact with a child almost daily, while 88% had at least weekly contact. The client population's functional status is indicated in Table 2 which presents dependency index scores for both clients and comparisons. Two important points need to be made concerning these data. First, for reasons discussed later in this paper, the scores show that the social service sites tended to recruit more severely disabled clients than did the sites under the auspices of health care providers. Second, the data indicate that the HCP is serving an extremely disabled population. Scores from the DMS-1, an instrument developed by the New York State Department of Health to assess eligibility for institutional admission to a skilled nursing facility (SNF) or health-related facility (HRF) (intermediate level), further indicate the extreme dependency prevalent among the treatment group. Scores calculated for the first 100 clients indicate that almost three-fourths of

Table 2

FUNCTIONAL STATUS BY GROUP

Dependency[a] Index	Clients (%)	Comparisons (%)	Site			
			CASC (%)	CFCC (%)	JSPOA (%)	FHC (%)
0	22.4	18.1	15	27	23	26
1	17.7	22.1	7	33	16	18
2	14.6	19.6	13	11	21	14
3	10.5	13.1	13	9	10	10
4	13.9	13.1	28	8	7	10
5	12.4	9.0	17	6	12	14
6	8.4	5.0	8	7	10	9
(n)	(474)	(199)	(137)	(105)	(108)	(124)
x̄	2.5	2.3	3.2	1.8	2.4	2.4

[a]The Dependency Index is a measure of dependency on six socio-biological functions: feeding, continence, toileting, transfer, dressing and bathing. Higher scores indicate greater dependency.

this initial group would have been eligible for either SNF (30%) or HRF (43%) placement.

Service Program

Available services. HCP provides three major services to its clients: (1) assessment, care planning and case management by an interdisciplinary team; (2) coordination of existing community resources, both health and social service; and (3) supplementation with critical gap-filling services.

Each of the four site agencies added staff to carry out client assessment and case management and to arrange with other existing providers for the services needed by the clients. Site funding covers an assessment team of a nurse, social worker and a physician consultant, two case managers and clerical support. The waiver services are provided through subcontract with approved homemaker agencies, pharmacies, ambulette, and taxi companies.

Assessment and case management. The assessment team makes a home visit to assess client status and service needs and to determine eligibility for the program. The assessment instrument elicits information from the client through a series of structured questions. After the in-home assessment which takes approximately 1-1/2 to 2 hours, the assessment team, the case managers, as well as a physician consultant, hold a planning session to develop a plan of care for the client. Utilizing the assessment findings as well as a "Physician Summary" completed by the client's primary care physician, the team formally completes a Care Plan, specifying client needs and the planned intervention to meet these needs. The process is repeated at six-month intervals for as long as the client remains in the HCP. The assessment and reassessment instruments provide the primary data for the HCP's research component.

The ongoing program component is case management. This includes arranging for services, either through another community program or directly through the Medicare waiver services. Follow-up and monitoring are major responsibilities of the case managers, who verify that services were actually received and that the client's needs are met. The overall status of the client is continuously monitored by the case manager and the assessment team nurse who makes visits in the home at least once every three months, in addition to the formal reassessment by the team each six months.

Funding and Financing Mechanism

Grants from HCFA and AoA covered the costs of ten full time project administrative and research staff at the New York City Department of Aging, as well as related expenses. Waivers were granted for the Medicare regulations which usually restrict coverage to those with acute, short-term skilled nursing or rehabilitative needs. The waivers cover client assessment and case management, up to 20 hours a week per client of homemaker and personal care services, prescription drugs and transportation to a variety of health and social service facilities.

HCFA's Office of Direct Reimbursement (ODR) served as fiscal intermediary for the project's waiver services. Bills for services were initiated by the sites, approved by HCP staff at the Department for the Aging and forwarded to ODR for payment. In the case of subcontracted services, the vendor (such as a homemaker agency) billed each site, which then followed the procedure previously described. A Periodic Interim Payment system, which allowed monthly advances to the sites based on approved budget, was developed by ODR to alleviate any cash flow problems.

The HCP's cap on personal care service at 20 hours per week per client served as the primary cost containment approach for the project.

RESEARCH AND EVALUATION

Research Design

In order to evaluate program impacts, the HCP is utilizing a quasi-experimental research design. A matched comparison sample of 200 persons from outside the project's catchment areas is being used, rather than a randomly assigned group. Randomization procedures, while clearly recognized as the optimal method in assessing outcomes, could not be incorporated in the HCP. The Department for the Aging, as a public agency and one which is mandated to serve as an advocate for New York City's elderly population, could neither ethically nor practically deny services to older people who otherwise met the HCP's eligibility criteria.

The original design called for the comparison group to be selected from recipients of Title 111C home-delivered meal programs who lived outside the geographical boundaries of the four sites and who otherwise met HCP eligibility criteria. However, due to the extreme levels of disability found within the treatment group (a somewhat unexpected outcome which will be discussed in the following section), it became apparent that initial comparison group subjects were significantly less impaired than were service recipients. Therefore, later comparison group subjects were drawn from the more severely disabled clients discharged from home health care agencies. Initial analyses indicate that this procedure has been successful in making the two groups more comparable in disability status.

At the HCP's completion all subjects will have been followed for at least one year, with many followed for as long as two and a half years.

Findings

Disability level. The HCP served a severely disabled population (see Table 2). This was somewhat unexpected, given the service limit (20 hours a week). Further, the HCP's target population was the unserved or under-served *community* residents—not hospital discharges or applicants to nursing homes—who might have been expected to have more extensive needs for in-home support.

Informal support. One important factor which can help explain the disability phenomenon is the relatively high level of informal support available to these clients. As the data in Table 1 indicate, family assistance was potentially available for the majority of clients.

Prior to receiving HCP services, families and friends were, in fact, extensively involved in providing both personal care and instrumental assistance. Of the total treatment group ($n = 504$), half of the clients reported receiving help from family members in bathing and dressing and approximately one-third had help in feeding (30%), toileting (36%) and transferring (32%). This help in personal care was generally provided on a regular basis. With the exception of bathing, almost all involved family members were providing *daily* assistance in these critical areas. Assistance with household and other instrumental tasks was received by even higher proportions of these clients. For example, more than four-fifths of all clients reported informal help in shopping (87%) and managing finances (83%); about two-thirds in meal preparation (69%), laundry (70%), light housework (62%), household repairs (65%) and filling out forms (68%); about half had regular help from family in heavy housework (50%), taking medication (44%), getting to the doctor (50%) and going outdoors (47%). However, the continued viability of their support without eventual assistance is extremely questionable. In fact, caregivers of 78% of the clients were judged by assessors to have a pressing need for respite. Therefore, HCP intervention was often targeted to providing support and supplementation for family efforts and the combined efforts of formal and informal providers enabled the HCP to enroll and maintain an extremely disabled elderly population.

Impacts. At the present time, efforts to evaluate the HCP's impacts are in the beginning stages and cover only the first six months of the client's life on the project. This period of time allows us to examine only the short-term consequences of an expanded service program. With this caution in mind, preliminary findings will be presented related to the HCP's impact on (1) hospitalization experiences, (2) institutionalization rates, (3) mortality rates, and (4) assistance from informal providers.

In general, HCP intervention does appear to have an impact on the client group's hospitalization experiences based on preliminary data from the assessment and first reassessment. During the year prior to initial assessment, 59% of the clients were hospitalized at least once, compared to 49% of the comparison group. The average length of stay per hospitalization reflects the somewhat greater frailty of the client group. Their length of stay per hospital admission was 16% higher: an average of 24.3 days as compared to the comparison group's 20.9 days.

However, the six-month follow-up revealed a major shift. While the proportion of each group hospitalized during this period remains constant, patterns regarding length of stay sharply diverge. The clients' average length of stay per hospitalization *declines* significantly by 29% to 17.3 days, while the comparison group experiences a non-significant 12% *increase* to 23.4 days. Clearly, the availability of a home care package, which can be mobilized in a timely fashion, is an important factor in explaining this major shift in hospitalization experience.

Preliminary institutionalization analyses cover all study participants for their first six months on the project. The rate of nursing home placements does not vary by experimental status within the short period of time covered by these analyses; 3.6% of the treatment group and 3.5% of the comparison group were institutionalized within their first six months of observation.

Similarly, mortality rates do not substantially differ within the first six months. The treatment group has slightly higher (but not significantly higher) death rates, with 11%, as compared to 7% of the comparison group, having died during this period. Since it is somewhat unrealistic to expect that home care services could have short-term impact on the risk factors associated with mortality, this early finding is more a further indicator of the clients' greater disability than a measure of program impact.

An important policy issue in providing long term home care is whether such services will result in additional health care systems costs by substituting for the care now provided by families. Very little empirical evidence now exists which addresses this issue. A preliminary analysis of the first 140 clients was conducted which compared presence and levels of informal support at assessment to that six months following receipt of services (Dono, Horowitz & Brill, 1982).

Informal assistance in ADL tasks (feeding, dressing, bathing, and transfer) was maintained over time. Assistance in toileting increased significantly from the baseline assessment to the reassessment (see Table 3). Assistance in ADL tasks responded to continuous daily needs that cannot be totally met within the homemaker's maximum allotment of 20 hours per week.

An examination of the 18 tasks grossly classified as IADL assistance also showed stability in informal support for most tasks. (See Table 3.) However, six tasks showed a significant informal support decline (cutting toenails, meal preparation, shopping, laundry, light housekeeping and minor repairs). These tasks' commonality is their boundedness, that is, they can be accomplished within a specific time period and, once accomplished, need not be repeated that day or week. Furthermore, most fall within the job description of the homemaker and can be accommodated within the time allotted.

However, the slight but significant reduction in the number of assisted IADL tasks (from 9.9 at assessment to 8.9 at reassessment) was found to be confined to a subsample. The reduction in informal assistance occurred only among the least disabled, the non-married, those living alone and those whose caregivers needed relief.

In summary, initial analyses suggest that the provision of expanded community-based home care services has a positive impact on length of hospital stay and does *not* replace the care provided by informal caregivers to any significant extent.

Table 3

PERCENTAGE OF CLIENTS REPORTING INFORMAL
ASSISTANCE AT ASSESSMENT AND REASSESSMENT

Task	Baseline Assessment	Reassessment	(n)
ADL			
Feeding	32%	36%	(140)
Toileting	30	44***[a]	(138)
Transfer	31	35	(139)
Dressing	52	51	(139)
Bathing	55	53	(139)
IADL			
Mobility			
Walking	16	29**	(140)
Get around the house	29	37	(140)
Up and down stairs	27	22	(139)
Going outdoors	46	44	(139)
Getting to doctor	42	36	(140)
Personal Care			
Shaving/combing	33	34	(138)
Cutting toenails	37	17***	(139)
Preparing medications	41	44	(138)
Household			
Meal preparation	72	60**	(139)
Shopping	83	71***	(139)
Laundry	70	42***	(138)
Light housekeeping	67	42***	(138)
Heavy housekeeping	59	61	(137)
Using telephone	43	44	(139)
Small repairs	82	72*	(135)
Picking up mail	69	66	(136)
Legal/Administrative			
Banking-bills	79	77	(139)
Filling out forms	73	73	(139)

[a]While the marginal proportions at baseline assessment and reassessment
are presented for ease of discussion, the McNemar Test which is used to
establish statistical significance is actually a test of turnover in the
cells representing change over time.
*p<.05
**p<.01
***p<.001

DISCUSSION: SERVICE AUSPICE, COORDINATION PATTERNS AND CLIENT CHARACTERISTICS

Several themes have begun to emerge related to service coordination by the four HCP sites. First, the nature and previous home
care experience of the agency had an impact on start-up and client
selection patterns. Second, all sites quickly reached their census

goals, found other community agencies cooperative, yet were unable to make extensive use of other community resources for their clients. Third, the HCP as a whole came to serve two particular subsets of the homebound elderly, namely, the extremely impaired with strong informal supports and the moderately impaired who do not have such support available.

While the HCP planners initially thought it desirable to have sites without extensive experience in traditional home health care, actual implementation experiences have indicated that a background in home care, with at least some community linkages already in place, is advantageous in the beginning stages of operation. It seems evident that the sites' experience prior to the HCP was an important predictor of how rapidly they would be able to carry out effectively the various tasks. Past relationships with social and health care providers within their communities tended to facilitate the processes of establishing interagency service agreements, subcontracts for waiver services and referrals of clients. Where these relationships were lacking the start-up time was delayed.

Related to this first observation is the recognition that auspice does influence the ease with which some start-up aspects can be handled. Our experience indicates that health and social service sites have differential strengths. For example, the health sites' previous ties with other health care providers as well as their previous experience in third-party reimbursement, enabled them to implement these program requirements rapidly. In contrast, the social service agencies' prior experience in providing in-home services and working with informal supports resulted in their early ability to attract and sustain at home a highly impaired client group.

Thus, each type of site had to complement its basic core services in order to meet the diverse needs of this homebound population. Staff at each site initially felt that the HCP represented a new direction for them. The health sites' staff saw the HCP as a social service program, while the social service agencies felt it was a health program. To compensate, the social service sites designated public health nurses as the HCP's lead team member, while one of the health sites chose to use a lead social worker and the other health site selected an administrator to coordinate the HCP.

Despite the fact that all clients met the same eligibility criteria, data revealed that client impairment levels varied from site to site. Contrary to original expectations, the two social service sites were admitting much more impaired clients than the health sites. Several possible explanations were explored and rejected, including the role of referral sources. Rather, it has become clear that the sites initially had different images of the kind of client who could be cared for at home within the HCP's 20 hour-per-week service limit.

The two social service sites both had several years' previous experience operating Title 111B home care programs. They knew that 20 hours a week of homemaker/personal care services, when coupled with informal supports, can be sufficient to care for quite seriously impaired clients.

On the other hand, the health care sites, although excellent ambulatory care providers, had no experience in home care. Although the health care sites had clear advantages in mobilizing pharmacy, physicians, and physical and speech therapies, they, like the social service sites, had a low percentage of hospital inpatients referred. This may reflect the health care sites' and referral sources' view that HCP services were not extensive enough to maintain a severely impaired population at home. The ambulatory health care sites initially accepted less impaired clients. However, one has now begun to admit much more disabled clients who have informal supports—clients they would have rejected 18 months ago.

None of the sites experienced difficulties in recruiting and maintaining its 100 client census allocation, and all four have extensive waiting lists. Three factors appear to account for this result. First, the HCP offered a service not available elsewhere, long term home care to a group above the Medicaid level. Second, each site was well established in its community with a variety of relationships with other providers. Both social service sites were lead agencies in coalitions organized around home care or aging issues. The two ambulatory health care sites had high community regard although they had not had the extensive service coordination experience of both the social services agencies. Third, each site had a contained catchment area which identified itself as a community within the City. One of these communities is actually an island (Staten Island) and site staff there feel that its forced containment facilitates interagency coordination.

Sites have not encountered any major resistance from other community agencies in their efforts to coordinate services for their clients. It seems clear that when a program offers service that was previously unavailable, other agencies are very cooperative because they want to have their clients admitted.

It was anticipated that the other community resources would be used extensively because of the limited HCP waivers. We found, however, that for the HCP's very disabled, above-Medicaid clients, there were very few existing services. Some of these services such as meals on wheels, friendly visiting and telephone reassurance overlapped with the homemaker/personal care services and the case management component of the program and could be incorporated into the 20 hours a week of personal care services without adding separate services. All sites were able to arrange with other providers for services for which reimbursement was available. Their effectiveness varied in obtaining services (such as physical therapy to maintenance level clients) where reimbursement was uncertain.

From the fact that all sites received many more referrals than their limited census would allow and continue to have waiting lists, it is clear that an extensive need exists for long term home care services among the currently Medicaid ineligible elderly. It also appears evident that the sites, when faced with many more client referrals than they could admit, had to choose the type of client who would best be served. In general, the sites eventually focused on the more severely impaired clients with extensive needs. The fact that such disabled older persons were found in the community points, as our data have indicated, to the presence of informal caregivers.

Overall, we have primarily attracted to the HCP two groups of older people: the extremely impaired with strong informal supports and the moderately impaired without close proximate caregivers. We can hypothesize that the relatively less impaired elderly with strong supports either do not request service or are not given priority for home care, while the needs of the extremely impaired without informal support exceed HCP capabilities.

Therefore, our client population's characteristics do not show that all seriously impaired homebound elderly can be maintained with the minimal service package offered by the program. We have clearly targeted (by outcome if not design) our services to a subgroup of the homebound elderly. The HCP could not handle and did not attract those disabled homebound without sufficient informal supports to complement homemaker activities.

Policy makers should be aware that although there are homebound elderly who can be effectively cared for at home with a maximum of 20 hours per week of formal services, there are many whose needs will require more extensive intervention. The agenda for the future requires that we make available and test a variety of service models in order to meet the diverse needs of this heterogeneous population.

REFERENCES

Cantor, M. H. et al. *Study of the elderly of the inner city of New York.* New York: New York City Department for the Aging, 1970.

Dono, J. E., Horowitz, A., & Brill, R. S. *The impact of expanded home care services on informal supports: Supplementation or substitution?* Paper presented at the annual meeting of the American Public Health Association, Montreal, November 1982.

Engler, M. *Title VII home-delivered meal program: A study of a selected group of participants.* New York: New York City Department for the Aging, 1978.

Health Systems Agency of New York City. *Home health care: its utilization, costs, and reimbursement.* New York: Author, 1977.

Health Systems Agency of New York City. *Health systems plan 1980-85.* New York: Author, March 1980.

Raphael, C. Testimony before the New York State Assembly Subcommittee on the Special Problems of the Aging Hearing on Monitoring the Delivery of Home Care Services, New York City Human Resources Administration, October 26, 1982.

Chapter 6

New York's "Nursing Home Without Walls": A Provider-Based Community Care Program for the Elderly

Dennis L. Kodner, MSP
Wilfred Mossey, DrPH
Rosina DeLuca Dapello, RN, MS

OVERVIEW

New York's "Nursing Home Without Walls" (named formally in its founding legislation as the Long Term Home Health Care Program or LTHHCP) is one widely discussed community care model aimed at controlling Medicaid outlays for long term care; increasing the availability of home care as an alternative to nursing home care; and removing barriers to the use of non-institutional services. The "Nursing Home Without Walls" program, proposed by Senator Tarky Lombardi, Jr., Chairman of the Senate Health Committee, was signed into law in August 1977 and became effective April 1, 1978. This statewide program became the prototype for the Medicaid Community Care Act (HR 6194), advanced by Representatives Henry Waxman (California) and Claude Pepper (Florida),

Dennis L. Kodner is General Director of Elderplan, Inc., Brooklyn, New York and Adjunct Assistant Professor of Health Policy in Medicine, Division of Geriatrics and Gerontology, Cornell University Medical College, New York, New York. Wilfred Mossey is Director of the New York State Long Term Home Health Care Program, Albany, New York. Rosina DeLuca Dapello is Director, Home Care Department, Metropolitan Jewish Geriatric Center, Brooklyn, New York.

The views expressed by the authors are solely their own and do not necessarily reflect the views of their respective agencies. Questions may be directed to Dennis L. Kodner, MSP, General Director, Elderplan, Inc., 910 48th Street, Brooklyn, New York 11219.

and ultimately enacted as Section 2176 of the Omnibus Reconciliation Act of 1981.

The "Nursing Home Without Walls" law is intended to create a
new permanent, statewide initiative in in-home care, rather than a
time-limited demonstration. In order to cover ten additional services
under the state's Medical Assistance Plan, Medicaid waivers were
obtained in October 1979, and, in conjunction with these, a four-
year project evaluation was funded by the Health Care Financing
Administration (HCFA).

The "Nursing Home Without Walls" program provides for the
establishment of individually-certified Long Term Home Health
Care Programs (LTHHCPs) in communities throughout the state.
Designed as the major entry point into a comprehensive range of in-
home and community-based health, social and environmental supports, LTHHCPs are primarily designed to serve Medicaid recipients who are "medically" eligible for placement in skilled nursing
homes (SNF) and intermediate care facilities (ICF).

LTHHCPs differ from more traditional forms of home care in six
significant dimensions: (1) all prospective Medicaid-eligible SNF/
ICF patients must be notified that LTHHCP care is an alternative to
institutional admissions where such is available in their area; (2) one
local designated *provider* takes responsibility for planning, providing and/or arranging, coordinating, and maintaining the appropriateness and quality of *all* skilled and non-skilled services; (3)
LTHHCP services exceed those Medicaid currently funds through
existing home care programs, including a wide range of psychosocial and environmental services available under a special waiver
from the federal government; (4) care is provided seven days a
week, with professional centralized management and coordination
available around-the-clock; (5) services are contingent on a multidisciplinary assessment indicating the need for institutionalization
and the level of care required; and (6) expenditures are capped so
non-institutional service costs do not exceed 75% of Medicaid costs
to serve the same client in the comparable institutional setting.

The combination of these elements creates a new type of community care organization which stands in contrast to New York's
existing Certified Home Health Agencies (CHHAs) and Personal
Care Service programs (called item 130 or Home Attendant Programs). These programs' benefits are limited: CHHAs provide
short-term medically-oriented care to mainly Medicare covered patients recently discharged from the hospital with active, post-acute

needs, rather than to the chronically impaired population with on-going, long-term needs; the Personal Care Service program is only able to offer non-medical home health aide, homemaker and house-keeper services over extended periods to assist with activities of dai-ly living. Furthermore, the CHHAs and personal care providers do not exercise full control and coordination over all aspects of patient care; are not available on a 24-hour basis; function within an open-ended, fee-for-service environment; and are not linked to a formal "gatekeeping" system.

Originally, nine sites out of 24 potential sponsors were selected to operate LTHHCPs with a total program capacity of 805 patients. As of March 1983, three years after the program's formal start-up, there were 32 approved LTHHCPs with a total patient capacity of approximately 3600 patients. Care is currently being delivered to more than 1,500 patients statewide, with more to be served as the twelve newest providers complete their pre-operational steps. More than 3,000 patients (not including readmitted persons) have been served since implementation, and there are currently 30 Certificate of Need applications from potential LTHHCPs in various stages of review and/or development.

In April 1982 the New York State Department of Social Services applied to HCFA under Section 2176 of the Omnibus Budget Recon-ciliation Act of 1981 to extend the program's waivers. Moreover, New York's newly-approved nursing home bed need methodology requires new LTHHCP providers be considered before additional SNF/ICF beds are approved in a particular area. As a result, "Nursing Home Without Walls" is now experiencing consolida-tion, accelerated enrollment, increased consumer and provider ac-ceptance, and growing recognition that LTHHCPs can effectively meet the needs of chronically impaired persons in need of long term care.

PROJECT ORIGIN AND OBJECTIVES

New York finances more home care services under Medicaid than any other state. Despite the magnitude of funding, State offi-cials have long felt that existing in-home services were poorly coor-dinated and largely unable to prevent or forestall nursing home ad-missions or assure frail older persons appropriate care to be able to remain at home. "Nursing Home Without Walls," though never considered a panacea, represents a major legislative effort to correct the various shortcomings in the state's extensive network of Certified Home Health Agencies and Personal Care Service Programs.

The legislation permits a mix of existing health care providers to operate LTHHCPs: Certified Home Health Agencies, SNFs/ICFs and hospitals. By allowing different providers to participate, the State can assess the relative strengths and weaknesses of each type of sponsor in meeting program objectives.

According to the State, there are five main objectives of the "Nursing Home Without Walls" program resulting from the original law, legislative amendments and State agency administrative directives:

- To provide an awareness about home care as an alternative/ forestaller to institutionalization;
- To reduce fragmentation in home care service provision to the elderly and disabled, and to demonstrate the effectiveness of coordinating and delivering such services through a single health care operator;
- To increase the availability and range of home health care services;
- To demonstrate that home care can be provided at a lower cost than institutional care to persons who qualify for admission to SNF/ICFs; and
- To show that home care can be effective in maintaining persons in need of long-term institutional care in the community when the necessary maintenance services are provided.

During the year following passage of the legislation (1977-1978), the State Department of Social Services negotiated Medicaid waivers and met with representatives of several other state departments and offices, the State Division of the Budget and the State Senate to discuss and resolve issues concerning reimbursement, client assessment, cost control, quality assurance, Certificate of Need and related programmatic areas. The existing administrative structure for Medicaid-reimbursed health services dictated the division of responsibilities for state and local development, implementation and monitoring of the "Nursing Home Without Walls" program. Figure 1 shows these responsibilities and complex inter-agency relationships.

During the implementation phase, the Department of Social Ser-

Figure 1

FUNCTIONAL RESPONSIBILITIES AND INTER-AGENCY RELATIONSHIPS

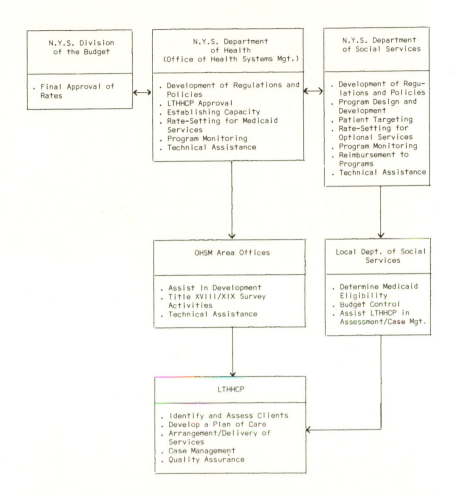

vices prepared and disseminated guidelines covering the referral process, eligibility and eligibility determination, notification procedures, assessment, case management, program implementation and rate-setting procedures for psychosocial and environmental services. The Office of Health Systems Management (OHSM) completed necessary revisions in the State Hospital Code governing operations of LTHHCPs; developed review and approval procedures for selecting initial LTHHCP providers; and processed

Medicaid reimbursement rates for traditional home health care services to be provided by the LTHHPs.

Between November 1978 (when the first LTHHCP patient was accepted) and late 1980 (when additional applications to become LTHHCPs were finally processed by the State), the program developed cautiously and slowly. The nine original programs served only 242 persons during the first year.

A number of factors account for this slow growth. First, numerous new policies, procedures and modifications of existing government practices and interrelationships had to be developed. Second, authority for legislative implementation and oversight was divided between two units of state government, initially with insufficient program staff. Third, apprehension in both OHSM and the Division of the Budget that "Nursing Home Without Walls" might increase public expenditures, rather than result in promised savings, led these agencies to treat the statewide program at first as a controlled, pilot project, setting capacity limitations on individual LTHHCPs that sometimes restrained further expansion. Fourth, early eligibility and assessment procedures were confusing and cumbersome, hindering program referrals and eligibility screening; further, misconceptions and misunderstandings about the LTHHCP target population and the program's unique patient care approach alienated many hospital discharge planners. Fifth, many potential LTHHCP clients were referred to other "competitive" Medicaid-reimbursed home care providers who were not hampered by the LTHHCPs' reimbursement limitations. Sixth, since the legislation did not fund planning and start-up activities at individual LTHHCP sites, little education about the new program or outreach to referral sources occurred on the community level. Seventh, State rate-setting and payment delays during the initial stage of development created severe cash flow problems, making existing LTHHCPs reluctant to expand. Finally, most LTHHCP operators delayed implementing waivered services, one of the program's most unique characteristics, because the State was late in implementing needed supplementary legislation putting necessary guidelines in place and providing special guidance on program development.

Between late-1980 and mid-1982, many of the problems impeding program growth were eliminated or diminished. A 1980 legislative amendment clarified the original legislation's intent, streamlined patient entry and assessment procedures and introduced greater flexibility into the patient care budgeting process. Integration of LTHHCPs into the State's Medicaid Management Information System (MMIS) and development of effective rate-setting and reimbursement procedures have minimized LTHHCP providers' financial problems. State activity to identify how the optional waivered services could be made available, utilized and reimbursed has led to an increase in their delivery by the sites and, therefore, greater recognition of the LTHHCP's uniqueness. Finally, as experience with the program among the referral network has developed, resistance from hospital discharge planners and other referral sources to the new client care perspective gradually is being overcome.

The program with the earliest success in enrolling a substantial number of clients was Metropolitan Jewish Geriatric Center (MJGC). MJGC is a two-site, 915-bed, multi-level long term care institution located in Brooklyn, New York. Brooklyn, one of New York City's five boroughs, is the home of one-third of the city's entire elderly population and has one of the most severe shortages of SNF/ICF beds in New York City. The LTHHCP is an organizational unit of the center's 386-bed Parshelsky Pavilion in Coney Island, a residential care facility with 96 SNF beds and 290 ICF beds. This voluntary, nonprofit organization is known as an innovative institution with a variety of inpatient and community services, including a day hospital, in-home electronic monitoring system, respite program, and research and community service arm. MJGC's willingness to meet changing community needs and to experiment with new health care delivery concepts is evidenced by its selection in Fall 1981 as the nation's first site for the demonstration of the Social/Health Maintenance Organization (S/HMO). The institution's positive experience with ''Nursing Home Without Walls'' was largely responsible for taking this new direction.

MJGC saw in the LTHHCP an opportunity to expand its functions and extend its services into the community. With the Center's designation as an LTHHCP operator, a comprehensive approach to geriatric care could be offered under a single provider umbrella. MJGC, then, had four principal organizational self-interests in applying to become a LTHHCP: (1) to meet identified community needs for non-institutional long term care services; (2) to ensure a role for the facility in what was perceived as a shift in the long term care system to community-based services; (3) to demonstrate that long term care institutions can operate community care programs; and (4) to provide the Center with a mechanism to extend its expertise, maximize the use of existing resources and change the mix of its patients.

MJGC submitted its initial application to operate an LTHHCP in June 1978, obtained State approval for a 100 patient program in November 1978 and admitted its first patient in May 1979. The original catchment area, containing approximately 110,000 persons age 65 and over in the Coney Island section, was expanded to include the central portion of Brooklyn, thus making the LTHHCP available to about 236,000 older persons.

MJGC's LTHHCP took about six months to develop operating policies and procedures; obtain reimbursement rates; secure and phase-in staff; negotiate provider service agreements; establish required transfer and referral arrangements with hospitals, long term care facilities, Certified Home Health Agencies, personal care providers and other local health and social service agencies; publicize the program; and create the advisory bodies required by law. MJGC rapidly expanded its patient enrollment and reached 90% of its certified capacity in about seven months in contrast to the slow, difficult start-up of most other LTHHCPs.

There are a number of reasons for MJGC's successful pattern of development. First, the Board and administration provided strong and continuing support, including the subsidy of over $100,000 in non-reimbursable funds. Second, prior to client enrollment, the program was fully staffed with self-starters having significant "hands-on" experience in home care of the elderly, thus saving time and preventing mistakes during implementation. Third, MJGC initiated aggressive outreach efforts, including ongoing involvement of community agencies in planning and implementing the LTHHCP; regular face-to-face contacts with hospital discharge planners; and use of a wide range of marketing techniques (from newsletters to television coverage, a telephone hot line, and presentations to local consumer and provider groups).

In August 1981, MJGC's approved capacity was increased to 150 and in November 1981 to 300 persons. During this expansion period the program reached certified capacity at times and, therefore, temporarily suspended outreach activities and instituted admission/readmission priorities and waiting lists. At the present time, MJGC has 300 active clients. Since May 1979, 618 individuals (not including readmitted patients) have been served, accounting for about 25% of all unduplicated clients enrolled in the entire "Nursing Home Without Walls" program since its inception.

PROJECT CHARACTERISTICS

Population Served

Initially, LTHHCPs admitted only clients who were: (1) financially eligible for Medicaid; (2) otherwise eligible for hospital care or placement in an SNF or ICF as predicted on the State's DMS-1[1] form; (3) seeking to remain in the community, with a viable home/residence in which to receive LTHHCP services; (4) able to have a care plan whose cost did not exceed the 75% cap discussed above; and (5) approved for participation in the LTHHCP by their personal physician and local Department of Social Services (in New York City, the Human Resources Administration). Although individuals of any age with chronic problems are eligible, the LTHHCP provides care mostly to persons age 65 and over.

After the first operational year, LTHHCPs were opened to private pay patients in an effort to delay depletion of personal financial resources and thus eligibility for Medicaid. Also, the 75% budgetary cap was clarified, applying it via an annualized rather than a monthly basis.

New York State has set priorities for client admission to the program in the following order: (1) dischargeable hospital patients requiring SNF care; (2) dischargeable hospital patients requiring ICF care; (3) dischargeable SNF patients; (4) dischargeable ICF patients; (5) community residents requiring SNF care; and (6) community residents requiring ICF care. To achieve these State admission priorities, hospital and long term care facility discharge planners mandatorily participate in the formal LTHHCP referral and assessment processes; the local Social Service Department is required to provide both verbal and written notification of all nursing home applicants concerning the LTHHCP option (the so-called "gate-keeping" mechanism); and targeted outreach efforts are undertaken by individual LTHHCP sites in their respective communities.

---

[1]New York State's DMS-1 assessment process, implemented in the early 1970's to classify nursing home levels of care, measures an individual's health and mental status and functional ability. Based upon a person's predicted needs for nursing care and therapies, a score is computed indicating the level of care. A score of 60-179 indicates a need for ICF care; 180 and above, SNF care. Total scores can be upwards of 2,000; individual LTHHCP participants scores have reached more than 1050.

Analysis of demographic characteristics of MJGC's 511 unduplicated clients served between May 1979 and September 1982 indicates that the average client qualifies for SNF care, is female, is age 77, has a circulatory problem, and was referred to the program from a community agency. She is likely to live with relatives (although 48% live alone) and is most frequently discharged from the LTHHCP to a hospital. Table 1 shows characteristics of MJGC's client mix through September 1982. The relatively high percentages of clients eligible for the SNF level of care (76%), discharges to the hospital (48%) and deaths (20%) confirm the view that individuals served by MJGC's program are seriously impaired and at high-risk of institutionalization.

Service Program

Assessment. The LTHHCP nurse coordinator and social worker, a case worker representing the local (county-operated) Department of Social Services, a discharge planner (if the client is hospitalized or already in a long term care facility), and the personal physician work as a team to assess the patient's health, social, psychosocial and home status; screen for admission; and consider Medicaid eligibility, service needs and budgeted costs for required services.

LTHHCP staff usually completes the DMS-1 form and carries out a home assessment. If the client is in a hospital or SNF/ICF, the discharge planner or floor nurse completes the DMS-1 form. The home assessment provides an opportunity to obtain a better understanding of the participant's and family's needs and to judge whether these can be adequately met by the LTHHCP in the home setting. Social Service Department case workers, also involved in the home visit, prepare the preliminary monthly budget based upon the plan of care developed by LTHHCP to determine whether the plan falls within the 75% cap on an annual basis. When the Social Service Department signs off, about 10-14 days later, the physician must approve the plan of care before services can begin.

Because complicated paperwork and difficulty in coordinating dual meetings can result in time lags, the State has developed an "alternate entry procedure." LTHHCPs may perform an initial assessment and commence services prior to the formal joint assessment in order to care for patients in need of immediate services. If the LTHHCP, however, admits a client who is later found ineligible, Medicaid reimbursement is retroactively denied. Since the

Table 1

BASELINE CLIENT CHARACTERISTICS
(May 1979 - September 1982)
(n = 511)

Age

Range	15 mos. - 104
Mean	77

Sex

% Female	73
% Male	27

Living Arrangement

% Living Alone	48

Referral Sources

% Hospital	30
% Community Agency	33
% Self/Family	26
% Long Term Care Facility	11

Reasons for Discharge

% Hospitalized	48
% Placed in SNF/ICF	10
% Died	20
% Improved	3
% Other (i.e., moved, personal reasons, etc.)	18

Average Monthly Budget ($) $1,023

Level of Care

Average DMS-1 Score	255
% DMS-1 Score of 180 + (SNF)	76

Primary Medical Conditions

% Circulatory	55
% Cancer	10
% Diabetes	5
% Musculoskeletal	15
% Respiratory	6
% Neurological	3
% Other	6

alternate procedure was instituted, MJGC has used it in about 80% of the cases admitted to the LTHHCP.

Clients are reassessed via the same joint process every 120 days (or sooner if the client's condition changes) to ensure that LTHHCP services continue to be needed and that the plan of care is up-to-date.

Method of case/service coordination. In the LTHHCP, case management is designed to match the client with prescribed services, ensure the delivery of an appropriate package of services from multiple service providers, and provide the client and family with a single, identifiable professional team to contact regarding any problems that might arise. As mandated by law, case management is available around-the-clock.

Case management and service coordination are theoretically shared by the LTHHCP and local Department of Social Services. However, as "Nursing Home Without Walls" has evolved, LTHHCP nurse coordinators and supporting social work staff have assumed total responsibility for day-to-day care planning, service ordering and coordination activities, service monitoring, quality assurance, and contacts with the patient and family. Social Service Department case workers, on the other hand, process Medicaid eligibility, monitor the budget and assist the LTHHCP in obtaining needed services outside the program's own formally linked delivery system.

Available services. An approved LTHHCP must offer directly or through contract all routinely-covered Medicaid services including nursing and home health aid services; laboratory and x-ray services; medical supplies, equipment and appliances; physical and occupational therapies; speech and hearing services; and personal care, homemaker and housekeeper services. A Section 1115 waiver enables providers to offer medical social services, respiratory therapy, nutritional counseling, home maintenance tasks, respite care, moving assistance, meals, social day care, social transportation, and housing improvement. Of the waivered services, medical social services, respiratory therapy and nutritional counseling are included in the State Hospital Code's definition of LTHHCP services and thus are mandatory. The other more socially-oriented supports are considered optional, but are provided by almost all LTHHCPs.

MJGC's LTHHCP provides the most comprehensive array of services in the state. These include physician visits, in-home and institutional respite care, home maintenance, housing improvement, social day care, social transportation, meals, an emergency alert response system for some patients living alone, moving services, consultation and support to terminally ill clients through hospice, medical day care, telephone reassurance and recreational services, and priority access to its long term care facility. MJGC coordinates both nursing home and hospital back-up for a smooth flow of LTHHCP patients among settings. Currently MJGC directly delivers physician care, some nursing services, rehabilitation therapies, nutritional counseling, social services, institutional respite and some social transportation, and contracts with community vendors for the other services. The LTHHCP has ultimate responsibility for prescribing services and maintaining their adequacy and quality.

Funding and Financing Mechanism

LTHHCPs are reimbursed by Medicaid through the traditional reimbursement system on a fee-for-service basis. Medicaid waivers, under Section 1115 of the Social Security Act, allow coverage of a wide range of services (discussed above) as well as the case management function. Flexibility is provided in defining what each waiver category covers, how the services are to be provided, and their costs. (For example, MJGC provides in-home electronic monitoring services under the home maintenance waiver.) Each LTHHCP's plan for waivered services must be approved by the State Department of Social Services, and some services (e.g., home improvements and home maintenance) must be prior authorized by the local Department of Social Services. As pointed out, funding for project start-up, and the cost of extensive outreach are not available as part of the program.

Expanding the LTHHCP's availability to "private-pays" has had an insignificant impact on the population served by the statewide program: only one LTHHCP provider has served private clients. This lack of service to private patients is probably due to the high cost of program services.

The "Nursing Home Without Walls" program contains safeguards against inappropriate service utilization: careful screening, planning and monitoring by individual LTHHCP's and local Social Service Departments, plus the State-established 75% expenditure cap. This annualized ceiling includes the cost of *all* medical services and treatments that the clients receive whether or not coordinated by the program. For example, if the local Medicaid reimbursement rate is $2,464 a month for SNF care, a patient requiring this level of care in the community in the LTHHCP is entitled to receive services costing up to $1,848 per month. In order to accommodate fluctuations in need, patients' individual monthly budgets can exceed this ceiling, as long as on an annual basis the total cost of care does not exceed the 75% cap. Large one-time expenses such as architectural modifications and the purchase of major medical equipment can be pro-rated over several months.

RESEARCH AND EVALUATION

From the Federal perspective, the "Nursing Home Without Walls" program is an experimental effort being conducted by New York State in cooperation with HCFA. An independent evaluator, Abt Associates, Incorporated (AAI) has been engaged to assess the program's impact and its potential replicability on the national level. This four-year research and evaluation effort, scheduled for completion in Summer 1983, involves the collection and analysis of health status, service utilization, cost and other significant data, including information derived from interviews with participants, family members, government representatives and providers.

The principal research questions are:

• What impact will the availability and use of in-home care have on the use of institutional services?
• What effect will home care have on the total costs and public expenditures for long term care services?
• How do in-home services affect care outcomes and clients' quality of life?
• How does the availability of coordinated funding and provision of in-home services influence the utilization of such care?

Research Design

The evaluation design consists of two components: a case study component of the nine initial LTHHCPs, and a quantitative component comparing LTHHCP patients and non-LTHHCP comparison groups. The case studies are designed to analyze program operations; assist in refining hypotheses and specifying analyses during the study's quantitative phase; assure accurate interpretation of data;

assist other sponsors interested in developing LTHHCPs; and evaluate the project's replicability. The quantitative analysis component has two sample groups, the LTHHCP sample and the comparison group sample, with approximately 700 individuals in each group. Both groups are being followed for one year with determinations being made of patient costs and service utilization for all health services (Medicare and Medicaid), costs and utilization experience of all other publicly-funded benefit programs (public assistance, food stamps, energy assistance, etc.) and patient outcomes. While there is no random assignment, the comparison sample group meet all eligibility criteria for participation in the LTHHCP; pass through the same points of identification (hospitals, nursing homes, community referrals, etc.) for participation in a LTHHCP but in areas where the program is not available; and meet the general age, sex, living arrangements, and disability levels of LTHHCP patients. In addition, the comparison areas were chosen (matched to treatment sites) on the basis of their distance from LTHHCP sites on a wide range of socioeconomic characteristics and health care system characteristics. The evaluator hopes to be able to utilize the quantitative data to compare LTHHCP and non-LTHHCP client behavior (outcomes) and allow evaluation of the extent to which LTHHCP substitutes for institutional care or provides augmented services for existing home care patients.

Findings

What has been learned to date? Based upon MJGC's experience and preliminary statewide evaluation data, we can conclude the following. First, the LTHHCP can effectively serve chronically impaired elders with severe multiple problems who presently meet the state's existing criteria for admission to an SNF/ICF. Second, statewide expenditures for the care of clients in "Nursing Home Without Walls" have averaged about 67% of the 75% cap or approximately one-half of the comparable cost of institutional care. For example, in 1982 the total cost of keeping clients on the LTHHCP was $13,592,192 (approximately). Institutional costs for the same clients over the same time frames would have been $26,987,156 (approximately). Therefore, the budgetary cap should not be viewed as a program impediment. Third, as determined through an interview survey of 40 LTHHCP clients and client families selected by the third party evaluator, clients and their families appear almost universally satisfied with the LTHHCP. The evaluator reports, "It is rare for the subjects of a study to almost unanimously agree that a program under investigation is the 'best thing to happen to me or my family'."[2] Fourth, data collected in the client interview survey indicate that the LTHHCP appears to have fostered an increase in informal supports and caregiving by family and friends. Finally, fifth, LTHHC providers who were not previously providers of home care (i.e., long term care facilities) seem to have been more effective in setting up and operating a LTHHCP in the initial years than were LTHHCPs based in Certified Home Health long term agencies or hospital-based home care programs (traditional home care). The long term care facility-based LTHHCPs were apparently more able to appreciate the difference in the philosophical approach of the LTHHCP as compared to traditional home care and operationalize it more quickly than others. Long term care facility-based providers increased the mix and range of services potentially available to clients, increased the number of clients served and increased their authorized capacity to serve clients. In addition, the long term care facility-based LTHHCPs seem to be more able to communicate these facts effectively to the referral network.

While the "Nursing Home Without Walls" program has experienced considerable growth and "success" in New York State, only a later analysis of program level cost and client outcome data will enable us to obtain more conclusive findings about the degree to which the program provides a cost-effective alternative to institutional care.

LESSONS LEARNED AND DISCUSSION: ESTABLISHING STATEWIDE COMMUNITY LONG TERM CARE PROGRAMS BY LEGISLATION

Despite intensive pre-operational activity, problems were bound to arise in such a complex statewide undertaking as New York's "Nursing Home Without Walls."

Start-up phase problems included difficult intra- and inter-governmental relationships; lack of staff on the state level; inadequate communications and information systems; cumbersome assessment

---

[2]See Howard Birnbaum, Christine Swearingen, Burton Dunlop, and Robert Burke, "A Case Study: Evaluation of the New York Long Term Home Health Care Program," Abt Associates, Incorporated, March 18, 1983, p. 105.

procedures; burdensome paperwork; poor understanding about the program's purposes, philosophy and patient care approach; limited outreach activities; absence of start-up funding; resistance from discharge planners; and poor cooperation between referral agencies and LTHHCP providers. As each of these problems was identified, solutions were fashioned through the combined efforts of State and local program administrators, LTHHCPs and interested legislative staff. The model that has emerged reflects a balance between the state's concern for programmatic and fiscal accountability on the one hand and the LTHHCPs' need for flexibility in serving the frail elderly population on the other.

The "Nursing Home Without Walls" program is still in an evolutionary stage. As experience is gained, consideration is given to modifying the original program design. Some of the changes that should be considered in the future are:

- *Expand LTHHCP services to include domiciliary care facilities.* Now programs can only serve clients in their own or relatives' homes.
- *Remove certain services from the 75% cap.* Services covered under the LTHHCP budget ceiling are supposed to be comparable to those under the SNF/ICF rate (excluding the costs of room and board). This is not strictly the case. Removal of non-comparable items like transportation and oxygen from LTHHCP budget consideration would provide greater flexibility in meeting chronic care needs.
- *Develop a family budget ceiling.* When more than one client in the household needs LTHHCP care, individual budgets could be pooled to maintain each in the community for as long as possible.
- *Further streamline screening and assessment procedures.* The "alternative entry" procedure allows LTHHCPs to admit clients without official authorization, but at their own financial liability by delaying the initial comprehensive home assessment. Consideration should be given to reduce further the time, complexity and costly assessment process by experimenting with a "waiver of liability" approach (like that in Medicare home care reimbursement) in which no financial liability occurs if a pre-determined proportion of denied claims is not exceeded.
- *Experiment with capitation approaches.* Consideration should

be given to providing LTHHCP services on a capitation basis thereby enabling a LTHHCP provider more flexibility in individual cases and not necessarily having to discharge a particular patient if his/her cost of care is slightly over the existing 75% cap. Another example could be to continue a LTHHCP within an HMO type framework. With the LTHHCP beginning to show an impact in terms of reducing hospitalization, the inclusion of acute care as an HMO benefit for an extremely impaired elderly population could demonstrate an impact on long term care costs. In addition, such an approach could contribute to greater integration and coordination of hospital and long term care services. One current example of this model is On Lok Senior Health Services. Another prototype under development is the Social/Health Maintenance Organization at Metropolitan Jewish Geriatric Center and three other sites nationally.

Although New York has the most extensive home care system in the country as well as longstanding involvement in the field, theoretically there is nothing in the program that cannot be transplanted elsewhere. In fact, New York's well-developed home care system was both a help and hinderance to program development. The program offers many interesting lessons to other states for creating community-based long term care programs:

- Appropriate organizational, professional and financial resources are required on the state level to mount community care projects, as they require considerable effort over long periods of time. States should cautiously introduce the program in order to minimize inevitable problems and make desirable changes.
- State-level authority should be consolidated as much as possible to plan, implement and monitor community-based projects. Designation of a *single* state lead agency with clear purpose and commitment should be encouraged at least during the start-up phase in order to diminish administrative fragmentation, communications problems and goal displacements.
- Community long term care programs should be carefully designed to ensure client access, cost control, quality of care, public accountability and sensitivity to the needs of front-line providers as well as clients and their families. Therefore,

systems and procedures should be free of confusion, undue complexity, costly duplication, and stifling bureaucracy. This especially applies to the assessment process.

- While uniform, statewide program design is necessary to define basic operational parameters, recognition should also be given to the uniqueness of communities and program sponsors and the need for flexibility in local program implementation and operations.

- The mere availability of reimbursement is not sufficient to develop non-institutional services and case management mechanisms. Government funds are also required for new community care providers' pre-planning, start-up, outreach and marketing activities. Rate-setting and reimbursement procedures for all community services must be established and operationalized before program start-up, as delay in fund flow can place local sites in financial jeopardy.

- Centralized data systems to monitor local project performance need to be in place prior to the program's implementation at the community level. This is crucial to the ongoing collection and analysis of accurate, current and comprehensive information on program utilization, costs and quality.

- Great care should be exercised by the state in the selection of potential community care organizations. In addition to evaluating a potential sponsor's ability to meet service requirements, consideration should be given to: the resources of the proposed sponsor; the organization's track record in long term care and aging services; the site's understanding of program aims; its political sophistication; and its sense of motivation.

- During start-up, the lead state agency should maintain ongoing liaison and effective, open communications with local sites as well as provide needed technical assistance. This will create a cooperative spirit and help to pinpoint problem areas as well as implement needed improvements.

- State planners and individual community care programs need to develop effective methods to target the hospital population, for the financial impact of older hospital patients awaiting nursing home placement is enormous. One of the most important approaches is sponsoring educational programs for discharge planners and other referral sources prior to and during local service delivery.

- Consolidated case management entities, wherein a single unit

coordinates *and* delivers most if not all non-institutional services, constitute a viable option in restructuring the long term
care system on the local level. Along with the freestanding
"brokerage" or channeling agency, serious consideration
should also be given to the use of existing, multi-purpose providers in fulfilling the coordinative/integrative function.[3]

The development of statewide community long term care programs as a result of legislation has its strengths and weaknesses. On
the positive side, legislation helps to make program goals and objectives explicit and institutionalizes the reform strategy. At the same
time, it establishes a formal framework for program development
and operations. Likewise, the program's legislative constituency
can be very supportive in facilitating desirable improvements and
fostering further growth. However, the legislative base can also be a
drawback, in that needed changes in the law require a great deal of
time and effort to achieve, even with the support of key legislators.

---

[3]For a more detailed discussion of this issue, the reader is referred to Dennis L. Kodner
and Eli S. Feldman, "The Service Coordination/Delivery Dichotomy: A Critical Issue to
Address in Reforming the Long Term Care System," *Home Health Care Services Quarterly,*
Vol. 3(1), Spring, 1982; and, Rick T. Zawadski, *On Lok Senior Health Services: Toward a
Continuum of Care,* On Lok Senior Health Services, San Francisco, 1979.

Chapter 7

Project OPEN: A Hospital-Based Long-Term Care Demonstration Program for the Chronically Ill Elderly

Lawrence J. Weiss, PhD
Barbara W. Sklar, MSSA

OVERVIEW

Project OPEN (*Organizations Providing for Elderly Needs*) is a research demonstration program designed to assess a coordinated hospital-based service delivery model in an urban setting. This long term care program provides an alternative to the existing fragmented health care delivery system. The program tailors services around individual needs, not upon third party reimbursement. Project OPEN offers to the population of "at-risk" chronically ill elderly a cost conscious approach to health care in which individual needs are assessed, appropriate community-based or home care services provided, and most importantly, independence promoted.

Project OPEN is just completing its fifth and final year of operation. As of June 30, 1983, the project ends it demonstration status. It is expected that the information obtained from Project OPEN will help evolve the long term care system at Mount Zion Hospital and

Lawrence J. Weiss is Research Director of Project OPEN and Barbara W. Sklar is Director of Project OPEN and Director of Geriatric Services, Mount Zion Hospital and Medical Center, San Francisco, California.

This research was supported by the U.S. Department of Health and Human Services, Health Care Financing Administration (HCFA) Grant #95-P-97231/9. The findings reported here do not necessarily reflect policies of HCFA.

Questions may be directed to Lawrence J. Weiss, PhD, Mount Zion Hospital and Medical Center, P.O. Box 7921, San Francisco, CA 94120.

127

Medical Center into a more controlled, alternative financial delivery system for the chronically ill elderly.

PROJECT ORIGIN AND OBJECTIVES

Project OPEN is operated by Mount Zion Hospital and Medical Center which for many years has seen the need for a coordinated and expanded service delivery system of health care for the chronically ill elderly. Mt. Zion has a long record of providing innovative health services to the elderly residents of San Francisco, having established, thirty years ago, the first west coast hospital-based home care program. During 1975, Mount Zion participated in an adult day health care demonstration program. The federal funding ended 18 months later but support from the hospital, private philanthropy, and now Medicaid reimbursement continued the service. The hospital also provides free geriatric health screening, a geriatric information, counseling and referral service, a life-line service, an in-home arts program, an adult social day center, geriatric medicine training fellowships, community health education, and a state-funded long term care demonstration program for Medicaid patients (San Francisco Multi-Purpose Senior Service Project).

Since Mount Zion Hospital has been an innovator in geriatric services and dedicated to providing comprehensive community care, the decision to establish a consortium of community health and social service agencies was a natural one. Hence Project OPEN began in October 1978 with a long term care research and development grant from the Health Care Financing Administration (HCFA), Department of Health and Human Services.

The project's first two years were devoted to planning and designing Project OPEN's consortium approach, its research endeavor, its organizational structure and its service components. Interest in and commitment to participate in a consortium approach were essential to the project. The consortium development planning phase involved assembling and meeting with staff from 18 provider agencies, then selecting and obtaining commitments from those who were to become consortium members. Consortium member selection was based upon: (a) population and area served, (b) existing service packages, and (c) reputation, flexibility and resources. The goal was to combine existing private and public sector service providers to develop a comprehensive, coordinated health and social service delivery system for the San Francisco elderly. Ultimately five agencies agreed to join with Mount Zion Hospital to form the consortium. These were:

- Kimochi, Inc. - a multi-service agency serving the Japanese elderly
- North of Market Multi-Purpose Senior Services - a multi-service health-focused agency in downtown San Francisco
- Laguna Honda Hospital - the county-run long term care facility which has intermediate, skilled and sub-acute inpatient bed levels of care
- San Francisco Senior Centers - a multi-site senior center providing recreational and social services.
- Western Addition Senior Center - a senior center serving the black community of the Western Addition

Services provided by consortium agencies, supplemented by other contracted agencies or professionals, were expected to enable the frail elderly to function at an optimal level of independent living.

While the consortium was being formed, the research plan, including evaluation tools, instruments and procedural protocol, was developed, and the organizational structure and service components were identified and defined. Partial implementation took place as well, during these first two years.

On August 18, 1980, Project OPEN was awarded Medicare waivers by the Secretary of the Department of Health and Human Services under the authority granted through Section 222 of the Social Security Amendments of 1972 (P.L. 92-603). As of that date, Project OPEN officially entered the operational phase of the program. The program is funded through September of 1983.

Project OPEN's overall objective is to design, implement, and evaluate a comprehensive long-term health and social services delivery system for a population of at-risk elderly. The program tests the ability of a consortium of service programs to provide appropriate, effective and cost-efficient care. More specifically, the program objectives are: to provide the necessary array of preventive and in-home support services in order to reduce the rate of institutionalization within acute care hospitals and skilled nursing facilities; to provide greater access to services; to maintain or improve the functioning levels of participants; and to maintain or reduce the total expenditures.

PROJECT CHARACTERISTICS

Population Served

Project OPEN's eligibility criteria are as follows: any person 65 years of age or older who has Medicare A and B coverage only (not Medicaid coverage), resides within a certain geographic area of San Francisco, and has health or social needs that make it difficult to live or function independently.

Project OPEN has a total client population of 338 clients: 220 demonstration participants and 118 control participants. Of the active demonstration and control participants, 55% are agency referrals, 17% are self referrals, and the remaining 28% are referrals from family members, friends or physicians. (See Table 1.)

The Project OPEN population mean age is 80 with its youngest participant 66 years old, and its oldest 99. Predominantly female (70%), the population is ethnically diverse, with 68% White, 19% Japanese, 11% Black and 2% other. With regard to marital status, 45% are widowed, 30% are married, 14% are single, and 11% are either separated or divorced. Although there are no economic criteria for admittance into the program, 70% of this particular population have annual incomes between $3,000.00 and $10,000.00. Overall, the population is comprised of middle and low-middle class community elderly that the project intended to target.

Service Program

Perhaps the most unique elements about Project OPEN are its systematic "step-wise" needs assessment, care plan development, service coordination, and regular monitoring of each demonstration client.

Assessment. A systematic functional status assessment is administered to each participant in the home by a Service Coordinator, who is either a public health nurse or a social worker. The assessment, which is administered in an interview format, includes: a brief personal health history, mental status, activities of daily living, instrumental activities of daily living, psychological status, social support and activities, environmental satisfaction, and physical status. This assessment serves as the initial indicator for a more extensive in-depth assessment (e.g., health screening, physical ther-

Table 1

BASELINE CLIENT CHARACTERISTICS BY GROUP

	Demonstration Group (n=220)	Control Group (n=118)		Demonstration Group (n=220)	Control Group (n=118)
Age			**Usual Residence**		
Mean (not %)	79.80	80.33	House	31%	20%
			Apartment (non-subsidized)	37	44
Sex			Apartment (subsidized)	25	31
Male	30%	31%	Room (i.e., communal)	5	4
Female	70	69	Residential/Personal Care i.e., Board and Care/ Senior Hotel)	1	1
Race			Other	1	0
White	69	66	**Living Situation**		
Black	10	12	Self Only	57	54
Japanese	19	19	W/ Spouse	26	28
Other	1	3	W/ Spouse and Others	2	2
Marital Status			W/ Child or Children	6	5
Married	31	28	W/ Others (not children)	9	11
Widowed	45	44	**Annual Income**		
Separated	1	2	$14,999+	9	7
Divorced	11	8	$10,000 - $14,999	14	19
Single	12	19	$ 7,000 - $ 9,999	22	21
Referrer			$ 5,000 - $ 6,999	26	21
Self	20	11	$ 3,000 - $ 4,999	23	26
Family	11	4	$ 1 - $ 2,999	6	6
Friend	5	8	**Primary Diagnosis**		
Physician	3	6	Cardiovascular	36	36
Agency	52	62	Gastrointestinal and Liver	5	5
Other	8	7	Genitourinary	4	3
Not Determined	0	3	Nervous System	6	8
			Bone and Joint	7	6
			Respiratory	7	10
			Arthritis and Rheumatic	14	8
			Other	21	24

apy evaluation) where appropriate. Reassessment occurs every six months or more often, as needed.

Care plan development. The assessment information for each person is summarized and presented at an interdisciplinary case conference. The interdisciplinary team consists of a nurse, social worker, physician, and other health professionals where appropriate (psychologist, physical therapist, occupational therapist, speech therapist). These professionals develop an individually tailored six-month plan of care for each participant that includes: a priority list of needs, the appropriate services, providers, locations, start date and the number of units of service recommended. Modifications and adjustments are included for the demonstration participants throughout the implementation of the care plan.

Service coordination. The implementation of the plan begins with the actual negotiation and participation of the client. The Project OPEN Service Coordinator contacts the designated service provider(s) and arranges for service delivery, i.e., the beginning date and the total amount of service to be delivered. Once the service delivery begins, the Service Coordinator continually monitors the client's condition as well as the quantity and quality of services received. This process includes consulting with the various providers to share information, to provide continuity, and to assure appropriate, quality care.

Available services. Project OPEN's scope of services is comprehensive, incorporating the traditional medical and health services provided through Medicare and private insurance, preventive services including monitoring and assessment, and social service provided through multi-purpose senior centers and in-home support services. Specifically, the following services are available from the consortium and other contractual arrangements: adult day health care; adult social day care; chore services; dental services; escort services; financial services; homemaker services; home health services; meals (home delivered); medical social service; medical appliances and supplies; medications; mental health services; outpatient medical services; podiatric services; rehabilitative services (occupational, physical and speech therapies); respite care; translation services (Japanese); transportation services; and visual care services.

Additional existing services available in the community which are not reimbursable by Project OPEN include: acute care services;

companion services; housing services; information, counseling and referral; legal aid; meals (congregate); outreach services; recreation; senior center programs; skilled nursing services; and telephone reassurance.

Funding and Financing Mechanism

Mount Zion Hospital and Medical Center acts as Medicare's fiscal channelling agent and authorizes the reimbursement of services provided by the consortium of agencies. Certain limitations and requirements within Title XVIII of the Social Security Act are waived by HCFA:

- *Waiver of duration, amount and scope of services* - allowing Project OPEN to cover the expanded services listed above.
- *Waiver of level-of-care limitations* - allowing payment for preventive care
- *Waiver of specific Medicare requirements* - allowing Project OPEN to forego co-insurance and deductibles as well as certain home care requirements.

Reimbursement for services provided under contract (i.e., consortium members and other contracted services) is made on the basis of negotiated prospective rates. Other sources of funding include private insurance, Older Americans Act money, United Way and other philanthropic monies, and individual client contributions. Even though Project OPEN is not able to pay for all services rendered to its participants, it does include tracking of the actural costs of all services rendered, discussed below under "Research and Evaluation."

Since one of the primary goals of Project OPEN is to provide cost effective services, several cost containment measures are used. Perhaps the most important approach is the Service Coordinators' actual functions of assessment, care plan development, and service authorization, which all contribute to cost containment. As a broker, the Service Coordinator negotiates with the providers for the appropriate amount of services, and then monitors the cost and frequency of services used. In addition, the Service Coordinator acts as an advocate and educator in facilitating a heightened awareness among the clients regarding service costs, bills, and third party statements.

Through Project OPEN's negotiated contracts with the consortium agencies and other providers, a reduction in service costs occurs. Since the project contracts for services and refers a greater volume of people to the contracting agencies, agencies compete for the project's business. The results are lower rates. Cost saving measures occur among private physicians as well, by encouraging the practitioners to accept Medicare assignment. All waiver reimbursement occurs on an individual needs basis and not on a third party regional paper review, or diagnosis basis. The result is an increased awareness of costs and cost containment decisions. In short, cost containment is maintained through Project OPEN's organizational structure and the design of the reimbursement system.

RESEARCH AND EVALUATION

Research Design

The project's research and evaluation methodology employs an experimental design, combining a randomized control group with a time series or pretest multiple post test method. The randomization takes place at the time of initial intake. Once a referral is made and the initial selection criteria are met, the person is randomized into a demonstration ($n = 220$) or a control group ($n = 118$). The demonstration participants receive the OPEN services (i.e., assessment, care planning, service coordination, and the benefit of extended reimbursable Medicare services) while the control group are tracked within the existing system of health care delivery and compared to the demonstration group. The longitudinal design enables research staff to observe the longer term impacts of the program for both quality care and cost issues.

The primary areas of analyses include functional status, care plans, service utilization and costs.

Findings

Our initial hypothesis concerning participant functional levels was that those in the demonstration group would maintain or increase their level of functioning over time, while the control group would decrease. The functioning levels and assessment of service needs of the participants were measured by the Functional Status Instrument (FSI) every six months. The FSI was designed to assess an elderly person's functional status in seven areas: Mental Status or orientation; Physical Status; Activities of Daily Living; Instrumental Activities of Daily Living; Psychological Status; Social Network; and Environmental Satisfaction. Seven scales were established and a total FSI score based on the summation of all the scales. Table 2 shows the results over a six-month period. A more detailed description of the FSI is in Weiss and Sklar (1983).

Although a longer period of time is needed before the full impact of the program on functional status can be evaluated, preliminary results (covering a six-month period) indicate that Project OPEN can prevent or at least inhibit the decline in functioning levels of those people with chronic disease. As shown in Table 2, demonstration group participants experienced only one significant decrease (Activities of Daily Living) out of the seven scales. The control group, however, showed significant decreases in two scales, Activities of Daily Living and Social Network, and in their total functioning score.

Another component of the functional data is the assessment of the participants' morale or level of life satisfaction. The expectation was that the demonstration participants will be more satisfied with life in general than the control group because they are participating in the project. At each assessment, morale was measured by a single question: "Taking everything into consideration, how would you say things are these days?" The participant is then offered the following possible responses: (1) Happy; (2) Both happy and unhappy, pretty happy, etc.; and (3) Unhappy, not too happy. The preliminary results, shown in Table 3, indicate that the demonstration participants who are unhappy at intake become moderately happy in the first six months. On the other hand, there is no change with the control group. The findings support the effective impact of the program on the participants' morale.

One final component of the functional data that needs addressing is the ultimate level of dysfunction—death. The mortality rate per client year for the demonstration group is 9% and for the control group is 7%. A mortality rate decrease was not predicted; however, the slight increase with demonstration participants was also not expected.

Another major hypothesis is that Project OPEN will provide effective health care to the elderly community. Effectiveness of care is assessed by the attainment of a specific measurable goal or service objective as projected in the care plan. At the end of each six-month

Table 2

FUNCTIONAL STATUS[a] BY GROUP OVER TIME[b]

Scale	n	Baseline Mean	6-Month Mean	t-Value
Medical Status				
Demonstration	165	4.85	4.82	- .22
Control	53	5.33	5.52	-1.35
Physical Status				
Demonstration	142	14.34	14.17	1.06
Control	38	14.32	14.98	- .61
Activities of Daily Living (ADL)				
Demonstration	159	17.83	18.51	-2.56**
Control	51	17.42	18.34	-3.25***
Instrumental Activities of Daily Living (IADL)				
Demonstration	137	22.36	22.71	-1.77
Control	41	22.17	22.66	-1.35
Psychological				
Demonstration	157	12.13	11.61	1.30
Control	46	11.25	11.65	-1.43
Social Network				
Demonstration	90	57.23	53.12	1.15
Control	28	58.23	59.02	-2.22*
Environmental Satisfaction				
Demonstration	159	8.32	8.01	3.17***
Control	48	8.35	8.20	.84
Total FSI Scale Score				
Demonstration	67	137.06	132.95	1.54
Control	15	137.07	140.37	-2.29*

[a] A higher score indicates lower functional status

[b] Functional Status Instrument (FSI) Scale Scores

* $p < .04$

** $p < .01$

*** $p < .002$

assessment period, the case conference team review the service goals. The results indicate that the demonstration group displays a significantly higher percentage of goals accomplished (74%) than the control group (34%) at the end of six months and at the end of 12 months (82% vs. 44%).[1]

---

[1] x^2(6 months) = 191, $p \leq .001$; x^2(12 months) = 96.8, $p \leq .001$

To increase the appropriateness of the health and social care within the OPEN delivery system is one of the explicit goals of the project. To measure appropriateness of care, services prescribed on the care plan are compared with those services actually received. The results to date show significant correlations between care plan service prescriptions and services actually received by both the demonstration and control groups at six and 12 month intervals. The mean number of matched services between care plan and services used during the first six months is 3.0 for the demonstration group and 2.0 for controls; at 12 months it is 2.8 and 2.1 respectively.[2]

Overall, the utilization patterns reflect that the demonstration group receives a more comprehensive range of services than the

Table 3

LIFE SATISFACTION

Life Satisfaction	Demonstration		Control	
	Time 1 Baseline	Time 2 6-Month Follow-Up	Time 1 Baseline	Time 2 6-Month Follow-Up
Happy	81	58	47	21
	(38%)	(35%)	(42%)	(42%)
Okay	74	81	49	23
	(34%)	(50%)	(43%)	(44%)
Unhappy	59	25	17	9
	(28%)	(15%)	(15%)	(15%)
Total	214	164	113	52
	(100%)	(100%)	(100%)	(100%)

[2] $\pm$ (6 months) = -5.34, $p < .001$; $\pm$ (12 months) = -3.06, $p \leq .01$

control group. The demonstration group actually receives an average of 6.4 services, compared to 5.4 by the control group.[3] The difference is particularly significant within the first six months where the demonstration used an average of 7.2 services the controls used 5.8. Specific demonstration group service utilization patterns reflect more frequent use of the waivered Medicare services (e.g., homemaker, transportation, day health care). Control group participants, limited to the existing institutional and medically oriented services, thus receive a less comprehensive service package, which costs more yet is associated with a decrease in functioning.

A major area of study for Project OPEN is the total cost of health, medical, and social care. The cost hypothesis predicts that the total cost of services provided to the demonstration clients is equal to or less than the control group. After approximately two years of program operation, a total of 3950 demonstration participant months and 1690 control participant months of cost data had been collected. Each service that the demonstration and control participants used was documented throughout the project. This was accomplished by talking with the participants and the service providers, obtaining bills, and obtaining the explanation of benefits from the fiscal intermediaries. The results shown in Table 4 indicate that total demonstration participant expenditures were 17% lower than the total control group costs. The average cost difference is $139.33 per client month or $1,671.96 per client year. These figures include the cost of service coordination ($41.10 client/month) and other extended Medicare benefits ($197.41 client/month). The savings for the demonstration participants occur primarily in the Medicare Part A or acute hospital services, where there is a $208.85 difference.

In studying the Medicare Part A Service Utilization, the demonstration group has an admission rate to acute hospitals of 36%, whereas the control group has a 48% admission rate (see Table 5). This 12% reduction in acute admission rate is significant. While statistically not significant, the acute hospital length of stay for the demonstration group averaged 2 days less than that for the control group (14 versus 12 days). The acute hospital readmission rate is 27% for both the demonstration and the control group.

Reducing the skilled nursing facility (SNF) admissions is another goal of Project OPEN. To date, there has been a significant re-

[3]F (demonstration-control) = 6.52; $p \leq .01$; F (time) = 3.57, $p \leq .01$

Table 4

COST SUMMARY
(August 18, 1980 to September 30, 1982)

	Average Cost Per Client Month				Average Difference Per Month
	Demonstration (n = 220)		Control (n = 118)		
Medicare Part A Services	$375.04	53.4%	$583.89	69.4%	−$208.85
Medicare Part B Services	73.39	10.5	120.71	14.3	− 47.32
Project OPEN Waivered Services	197.41	28.1	113.88	13.5	+ 83.53
Other Non-Waivered Services	15.18	2.2	22.97	2.7	− 7.79
Service Coordination	41.10	5.8	-0-	-0-	+ 41.10
TOTALS	$702.12	100%	$841.45	100%	−$139.33

duction in the SNF admission rate as shown in Table 5: 6% for the demonstration group as compared to 8% for the control group. The average number of SNF bed days for the total sample does not differ significantly (13 days for the demonstration participants, 17 days for the control group), but, along with the SNF admission rate decrease, probably contributes to the cost savings for the demonstration participants. However, since the numbers admitted to SNF's are small, in part due to the project's intake design, no conclusive statements about SNF utilization can be made at this time.

In sum, Project OPEN's preliminary results reflect improvements in the demonstration group's functioning, morale, service comprehensiveness (variety of services utilized), goal accomplishments, and the appropriateness of services. In addition, the results indicate a decrease for the demonstration group in actual costs and in acute hospital and SNF utilization as compared to the control

Table 5

INPATIENT SERVICE UTILIZATION
(August 18, 1980 to September 30, 1982)

Type of Facility	n	Percentage of Users	No. of Inpatient Days	No. of Inpatient Days Per Total Sample	No. of Episodes Per Hospital Client	Average Days Per Episode	No. of Hospitalized Patients Readmitted
Acute Hospital							
Demonstration	220	36%	1670	8	1.8	12	38 (48%)
Control	118	48%	1413	12	1.8	14	28 (49%)
Skilled Nursing							
Demonstration	220	6%	2811	13	0.8	216	--
Control	118	8%	1947	17	2.1	216	--

group. These findings indicate that the project is meeting most of its original objectives and perhaps can serve as an alternative hospital-based health service delivery model for the chronically ill elderly.

LESSONS LEARNED

The experience gained in Project OPEN has several implications for future development of comprehensive long term care policy. First, it is apparent that there must be a focus on long term care services at the national and state level. Second, that there should be flexibility in design of the local delivery system, enabling local communities to decide what is most appropriate to their particular environment. Third, Project OPEN's results argue for the connection of long term care services with the acute care system and for the inclusion of cost-effective nontraditional services among those reimbursed under Medicare and Medicaid. Assessment, service coordination or case management, and maintenance and prevention services should be the basis for the service delivery system.

Project OPEN's population appears to be less functionally impaired than the demonstration participants in other projects. In developing long term care systems, therefore, it may be appropriate to target a slightly healthier population than those who require a 24-hour skilled nursing level of care. By intervening earlier in the process of chronic disease and by targeting elderly persons who are at-risk of needing more dependent levels of care, both 24-hour care and acute hospital care can be delayed or even avoided.

DISCUSSION: THE HOSPITAL'S ROLE IN THE DELIVERY OF LONG TERM CARE SERVICES

Project OPEN is a unique long term care demonstration program, the only hospital-based demonstration program in the country that provides such a comprehensive range of services to the chronically ill elderly. The hospital-based long term care system has both advantages and disadvantages as seen from the Mount Zion perspective. These advantages and disadvantages may be discussed from the vantage point of the system, community agencies serving the elderly, the hospital, and the patients or participants.

A few acute care hospitals have a history of providing the elderly with special services. For example, the Philadelphia Geriatric Center in Pennsylvania provides a variety of independent living projects in conjunction with their geriatric hospital. In 1947, Montefiore Hospital in New York City extended their services to include home health care. More recently, chronic care services such as "swing beds," telecare, adult day health care, geriatric assessment and screening, hospice, etc. are being incorporated into the acute care hospital's structure. Outreach programs establishing more community linkages are becoming more frequent, but according to Evashwick (1982) only 18% of the 417 hospitals she surveyed had outreach programs and 25% (or less) of the sample had special services for the elderly. Only the following services were offered by more than 25% of the hospitals: discharge planning (76%), information and referral (48%), patient education (43%), skilled nursing facility care (39%), and psychosocial counseling (31%). All other special services were provided by a very small proportion of hospitals: mental health services (23%), home health care (22%), comprehensive assessment (9%), and outpatient rehabilitation (9%). Clearly, the general hospital can provide multiple services to the elderly and chronically ill, but this expanded role is in its infancy.

A distinct advantage that hospitals have over other community agencies in serving long term care patients is that they are fairly secure organizations with many resources, materials, and knowledgeable professionals upon which to draw. The extent of the resources include fiscal and cash flow advantages, an established organization of volunteers, management and legal personnel, accounting and data processing systems, a broad political power base, and, perhaps most important, access to numbers of chronically ill elderly. Entry into a long term care system is a critical issue and hospitals can provide the doorway to a target group of elderly that are at-risk of needing more dependent services.

Mount Zion Hospital has the reputation within the community as an innovator in geriatric services and as a caring institution. Thus, other agencies as well as the medical community accepted and participated in the design of Project OPEN. Knowledge about health care, reimbursement and fiscal issues is vital to community agencies in identifying service and program costs and Mount Zion's assistance in developing better fiscal and documentation techniques solidified its relationship with community agencies. Another advantage to the community agencies of a hospital-based system is the potential for more collaborative social, health, and medical services. Through the development of a working collaborative consortium of services, each agency's political base can be broadened. Social services become more recognized and acceptable to the medical community, while the social service workers develop a greater understanding of medical procedures and practices. The medical, health, and social service disciplines educate each other, making possible a comprehensive assessment of the patient's needs and a plan of care. The expected result is an increase in the effectiveness of patient care.

The patients or participants in a hospital-based system of long term care are more accepting of social and mental health services because they are subsumed under the rubric of medical services. Since medical services are more respected and accepted by the elderly, programs associated with a medical institution are used to a greater degree than those of a social service agency. This attitude difference has been found at Mount Zion. When comparing Mount Zion's utilization patterns with those of a nearby family service agency, it was discovered that the elderly needing social services preferred Mount Zion Hospital over a neighboring service agency, based on several clients' expressed attitudes.

In addition, when participants in a hospital-based long term care system need medical care, the service coordinator (a hospital employee) knows the institution and its processes, thus is more able than a person from outside the hospital to access the needed services. Constructive use of the hospital's knowledge and the medical procedures can help relieve anxiety and stress experienced by patients due to hospitalizations. Advocacy and education around medical problems and treatment procedures are also performed by the service coordinator in the hospital setting. The result is an increase in compliance within the hospital and cooperation outside the hospital. Quality care issues can be directly affected by such a hospital-based long term care system as modeled by Project OPEN.

Providing a comprehensive long term care system such as Project OPEN offers several advantages to the hospital. Referrals to the hospital are generated due to the array and quality of services available. Revenues to the many departments within the hospital are produced by increasing the patient population and revenue sources are diversified. A reduction in the utilization of hospital administrative days results from the service coordinators' knowledge of the patients, the home environment and support system. The discharge planning function is largely performed by the service coordinators because of their thorough knowledge of the client and community resources. Staff problems with patients within the hospital are minimized by having comprehensive information about the patient's total condition and a professional service coordinator to mediate any difficulties. An increase in communication between physicians, nursing staff, and patients leads to increased treatment cooperation and more efficient use of hospital personnel.

Promoting the health team concept is an important component of the chronically ill patients' treatment plan. By placing the long term care system within the hospital setting, an educational process occurs with the medical profession. Physicians learn to listen to other health professionals and make collaborative decisions regarding patient care. This inter-disciplinary cross fertilization not only educates physicians, but all other health and social service staff benefit from the educational process.

One additional advantage to the hospital of incorporating a long term care system is the establishment of a comprehensive patient data Information Management System (IMS). Project OPEN's IMS has provided Mount Zion's hospital administration with a method of monitoring and reporting on patient utilization, cost, and functional status information on program participants. This information aids management in planning and decision making for future operations. A hospital's existing data processing resources coupled with an attitude of providing patient coordination and continuity of care can greatly facilitate the development of a comprehensive system of health care for the elderly.

The disadvantages of being a hospital-based system are costs, traditional focus on acute medical treatment, and institutional layers of bureaucracy. Somers (1982) discusses the disadvantages of higher costs set up for hospital accounting. Because of the established Medicare and Medicaid formulas for allocating costs across hospital departments, programs may need to pay for costs of line items with which they have no relationship, utilization, etc. Program administrative and service costs in a hospital setting are clearly higher than in freestanding service agencies. Unfortunately, geriatric service overhead expenses (whether for service coordination or home care) take into consideration other hospital support services and equipment.

A second disadvantage is that hospitals traditionally have been in the business of acute care and medical treatment. However, a long term care program necessitates changing the milieu to look at the delivery system in new and different ways. In addition to the traditional acute care that is provided in the hospital, rehabilitative maintenance and preventive services are needed. Traditional facilities have a tendency to resist change. Therefore, the hospital's board, administrative personnel and medical staff must support philosophically and programmatically the provision of expanded services to the the the chronically ill elderly.

Another disadvantage to a hospital-based system lies in the institutional layers of bureaucracy. For example, a simple intake form needs to be processed through time consuming channels in order to be approved for use. Staffing patterns and demands are constrained by the fact that the hospital is a health facility subject to various licensing requirements. More flexibility in staffing and management might exist if the program were not hospital-based.

No one health or social facility provides the optimum environment for the lead agency in long term care. The hospital-based system as discussed from Mount Zion Hospital's (Project OPEN) perspective presents distinct advantages and disadvantages. The development and nature of services depend on the hospital environment, philosophical commitment and support from its administration, board, medical staff, and community agencies. In Project OPEN's experience, the advantages of the hospital-based system have far outweighed the disadvantages.

REFERENCES

Evashwick, C. Long term care becomes major new role for hospitals. *Hospitals,* 1982, *56,* 50-55.

Skellie, F. A., & Coan, R. E. Community-based long term care and mortality: Preliminary findings of Georgia's Alternative Health Service project. *The Gerontologist,* 1980, *20,* 372-379.

Somers, A. Moderating the rise in health care costs. *New England Journal of Medicine,* 1982, *307* (15), 944-947.

Weiss, L. J., & Sklar, B. W. An alternative health delivery system for the chronically ill elderly. *Prevention in Human Services* (Volume 3:1). New York: Haworth Press.

Chapter 8

On Lok CCODA:
A Consolidated Model

Marie-Louise Ansak, MSW
Rick T. Zawadski, PhD

OVERVIEW

On Lok Senior Health Services' Community Care Organization for Dependent Adults (the CCODA) is a consolidated, community-based long term care program. Through the CCODA On Lok provides *all* health and health-related services needed by its frail elderly population—from acute hospitalization to transportation, translation, home-delivered meals and recreation therapy. Thus the CCODA differs from both brokerage/channeling and traditional long term care approaches in that: (1) the full range of social and medical services are integrated into a single health program; (2) services are delivered by the same professionals planning them; and (3) there exists an opportunity and implicit financial incentive to control costs with total control over all expenditures.

The CCODA represents a third phase in the development of On Lok's health program for the elderly of San Francisco's Chinatown-North Beach-Polk Gulch area. On Lok is one of the oldest community-based long term care programs. In the early 1970's, the program was funded to develop a single day health center. A few years later,

Rick T. Zawadski is Research Director and Marie-Louise Ansak is Executive Director, On Lok Senior Health Services, San Francisco, California.

The CCODA service program was supported by waivers granted by the USDHHS Health Care Financing Administration (#95-P-97234) under Section 222 of P.L. 92-603. The research and development was supported by grants from the Office of Human Development Services (#18-P-00156/9), the Administration on Aging (#18-P-00156/9), The National Institute for Handicapped Research (#12-P-59368/9), United Way of the Bay Area, and private contributions. The views expressed in this paper are those of the authors. Questions may be directed to Rick Zawadski, On Lok Senior Health Services, 1455 Bush Street, San Francisco, CA 94109.

147

the program expanded to provide a range of outpatient and in-home services. In 1978, with funding from the Office of Human Development Services and Medicare waivers, the CCODA was begun and has since developed into a comprehensive program serving nearly 300 older people, all of whom have been certified (by a state Medicaid representative) as eligible for institutional care.

Beginning in 1983, On Lok will shift its CCODA from single source funding (Medicare) to a mix that reflects cost responsibility under the traditional system (that is, to include Medicaid, private insurers and individual co-payments as well as Medicare). In so doing, On Lok will also become the first community long term care provider to assume some risk for the cost of long term care.

PROJECT ORIGIN AND OBJECTIVES

On Lok Senior Health Services, which operates the CCODA, is a freestanding, nonprofit community-based organization. It was incorporated in 1971 to provide quality long term care to frail older people living in San Francisco's Chinatown-North Beach area. In addition to its service program, On Lok has a research unit and a technical assistance arm known as On Lok Institute. A separate corporation, the On Lok Development Corporation, operates On Lok House, a 54-unit HUD 202 Project. On Lok Senior Health Services' CCODA provides services to program enrollees in a variety of locations: most frequently in one of its three adult day health centers (one of which is located on the premises of On Lok House), but also in participants' homes and in acute care hospitals and nursing homes under contract with On Lok.

On Lok began through the efforts of a community group that, in 1966, was seeking a better solution to the long term care needs of the area's elderly. At that time, the only options available to the Chinatown-North Beach elderly—many of whom spoke little or no English—were fragmented community services or institutionalization a long way from home, where no one spoke the older persons' language. Although the original plan was to build a nursing home in the community, the group decided instead to establish a day center based on the English model. Via a grant from the Administration on Aging in 1972, On Lok developed a multi-level, multi-purpose day center (Kalish, Lurie, Wexier and Zawadski, 1975).

With support from Medi-Cal (California's Medicaid) demonstration contracts, On Lok became the prototype for California's adult day health service and played a role in making adult day health a legislated Medi-Cal benefit (RTZ Associates, 1977; Von Behren, 1979). Next, via a model project grant from the Administration on Aging (1975-79), On Lok expanded its day center program to encompass an outpatient continuum of health services (in-home chore, portable meals, housing assistance, and social level day care). A multidisciplinary team coordinated all services (Zawadski, 1979).

In 1978, On Lok launched its CCODA effort with a research grant from the Office of Human Development Services. By 1979 the entire outpatient system, including primary medical care, was operational with Medicare waivers covering all services. By 1980 the inpatient components had been added to complete the system. The CCODA's five objectives were: (1) to develop and operate a centrally funded and administered community care system; (2) to assess the impact of prospective, capitated, decategorized funding on service utilization, quality and cost; (3) to contrast the management efficiencies of the CCODA model with those of presently operating long term care approaches, including brokerage models; (4) to develop actuarially sound methods of budgeting to meet the needs of dependent adults; and (5) to produce a cost and utilization yardstick by which to measure the effectiveness of other service models.

PROJECT CHARACTERISTICS

Population Served

On Lok's CCODA, by design, serves an institutionally-certified elderly (55 and over) population. When the CCODA began, participants from On Lok's previous program were allowed to join regardless of their current institutional eligibility status (that is, they were grandparented into the CCODA). Of those grandparented into the program, almost all were certified for institutional care at the time they joined On Lok and many remain eligible for such care. All new CCODA participants are admitted only if they meet state criteria for care in a skilled nursing or intermediate care facility.

All CCODA participants must reside in On Lok's approximately four square mile catchment area—an area with 18,230 people over the age of 65, according to the 1980 census. About 40 people are referred each month for admission to the program with only about six ultimately enrolled. Most are rejected because they are not sufficiently impaired or do not reside in the geographic area. Table 1 provides baseline demographic and functional status information for

Table 1

BASELINE CLIENT CHARACTERISTICS

	n	%
Age	449	
Below 64		6
65 - 74		26
75 - 84		47
85 or above		21
Sex	449	
Male		54
Female		46
Ethnicity	449	
Chinese		73
Caucasian		14
Filipino		5
Italian		5
Hispanic		2
Black		<1
Other Asian		<1
Other		<1
Marital Status	449	
Single		15
Married		28
Widowed, Divorced, or Separated		57
Primary Language	446	
Chinese		72
English		18
Tagalog		4
Italian		4
Spanish		2
Other		<1
English Fluency	446	
None		33
Little		27
Fair		15
Fluent		25

Table 1 (cont'd)

	n	%
Source of Income[a]	430	
SSA		76
SSI		45
Pension		15
Investment		1
Family Support		1
Other		5
Medicare Eligibility	449	
Medicare/Medicaid		44
Medicare Only		48
Medicaid Only		3
None		5
Cognitive and Bodily Impairments		
Long-Term Memory	443	62
Short-term Memory	443	69
Orientation	440	44
Reasoning	441	49
Attention Span	442	40
Vision	420	81
Hearing	430	61
Speech	426	18
Upper Extremity	430	56
Lower Extremity	426	74
Bladder	422	35
Bowel	420	32
Activities of Daily Living		
Eating	426	9
Dressing	425	36
Grooming/Hygiene	424	49
Bathing	426	65
Toileting	423	27
Cooking	420	77
Shopping	425	75
Home Chore	418	78
Laundry	422	76

Table 1 (cont'd)

	n	%
Primary Medical Diagnosis	440	
by ICDA Category		
Infectious/parasitic		2
Neoplasm		3
Endo/Nutri/Metabolic		11
Blood/Blood Forming		<1
Mental Disorder		11
Nervous System (Stroke)/Sense Organ		28
Cardiovascular		24
Respiratory		4
Digestive		3
Genitourinary		3
Skin		1
Musculoskeletal		6
Congenital		<1
Accidents/Poisoning		2
Ill-Defined		3

Note. For participants admitted into the CCODA program from February 1972 through June 1982.

[a]One or more sources cited

program participants admitted from February 1979 through June 1982 (including 146 grandparented into the CCODA).

During the first quarter of 1983 (January - March), monthly program enrollment averaged 288 participants. These participants' characteristics were similar to the baseline characteristics displayed in Table 1. Of these, nearly all (263 or 93%) were Medicare-eligible. Their average age was 79 and females slightly outnumbered males (51% versus 49%). Most participants received income from Social Security (75%), nearly half (49%) received SSI, and about one-sixth (16%) had investment income; their average monthly income was $534. Compared with the baseline statistics shown in

Table 1, the ethnic mix remained about the same. However, more were cognitively impaired, fewer had vision (52%) or hearing (44%) impairments and more had ADL impairments. Their primary medical diagnoses were about the same as those shown in Table 1, with diseases of the nervous and cardiovascular systems predominating. Participants continued to average five medical diagnoses each.

Service Program

Assessment and coordination. All participants receive a comprehensive evaluation of their medical, functional, and psychosocial status by On Lok's multidisciplinary intake and assessment team which consists of a physician, nurse, social worker and physical/occupational therapist. Services are authorized by the team based on this multidisciplinary assessment. Participants are reassessed regularly, either at six-month or three-month intervals, depending on health and functional status. The intake and assessment team functions together as the case manager. With respect to service coordination, the social worker plays the key role, acting as the person's counselor and advocates both within the program and outside of it, for example, with family matters, personal finances, and housing.

Available services. Services are provided directly by On Lok staff (or under contract, directed and supervised by On Lok staff) and usually by members of the intake and assessment team. On Lok's service team includes physicians, nurse practitioners, social workers, a dietician, nurses, physical therapists, home care attendants, licensed home health aides, occupational therapists, recreational therapists, drivers, and health workers. Part-time On Lok staff includes medical specialists (optometrist, dentist, psychiatrist, podiatrist, audiologist) and contracted services include acute hospital care, skilled nursing care, medications, laboratory testing, x-rays, inpatient medical specialty services, restorative and supportive appliances and emergency medical transportation (see Figure 1).

Services which may be authorized for On Lok participants include medical services such as physician and pharmacy consultant services, rehabilitative services such as physical and occupational therapy, social services such as medical social services and activity services, and supportive services such as dietary services (Chinese, Western regular or special diet meals at center or home-delivered, dietary counseling), transportation (nonemergency to and from cen-

Figure 1

SERVICES PROVIDED THROUGH THE CCODA PROGRAM

BY ON LOK STAFF	BY PART-TIME ON LOK STAFF
- Primary physician services - Skilled nursing care, including medications - Physical, occupational, speech and recreational therapies (group and individual) - Social casework services (including financial management) - Nutritional counseling and educ. - Meals (both congregate and home-delivered with special diets--Chinese and Western menus) - Transportation (to and from centers and for other non-emergency services) - Adult day health - Personal care - In-home attendant/homemaker services - Home health care - Discharge planning - Hospice care - Case management	- Primary physician (weekend, evening and backup services) - Optometry - Audiology - Dentistry (including dentures) - Psychiatry - Podiatry BY CONTRACT - Acute hospital care - Skilled nursing care - Drugs, medications - Laboratory testing - X-rays - Inpatient medical specialty services - Restorative and supportive appliances - Emergency medical transportation

ters, outpatient facilities and other providers as well as emergency services), and health worker services (rehabilitation aide, personal care, homemaker, escorting and interpreting services). All contracted services listed in Figure 1 may also be authorized for participants.

Funding and Financing Mechanism

The On Lok CCODA service program is funded primarily by Medicare waivers under Section 402(b) of the Social Security Amendments of 1967 (as amended by Section 222 (b) (1) of P.L. 92-603). Waivers have permitted payment of cost with prospective interim payments based on estimated capitation rate rather than service units. They have allowed total reimbursement through Medicare for all inpatient and outpatient, health and health-related services provided through the CCODA. The waivers included:

- removal of all Medicare service restrictions and limits;
- liberalization of Medicare entitlement requirements;
- inclusion of normally uncovered medical specialties (e.g.,

dentistry, pharmacy), supportive and preventive services;
- dispensation from traditional review and reporting requirements; and,
- elimination of all participant co-insurance and co-payment responsibility.

For most of the services not provided directly by On Lok staff (e.g., pharmacy, laboratory and x-ray services), On Lok negotiates fixed rate contracts (usually the Medi-Cal rate plus 10%). For acute hospital and skilled nursing care, On Lok contracts with two hospitals and one nursing facility, using an all-inclusive per diem rate. The same form is used by the On Lok team in authorizing contracted services and by the contracting providers to bill On Lok for these services.

While the program has been reimbursed for its costs, prospective capitation reimbursement with the assumption of risk has been an objective. On Lok's total control over all expenditures has provided the opportunity to contain health care costs. Knowing that the survival of its "ideal" system depended on its costs being the same or lower than the traditional system's gave On Lok the opportunity and implicit incentive to control costs. With the new demonstration, the incentive will be explicit for On Lok will share the risk with its funders.

The CCODA research has been supported by the Office of Human Development Services, the National Institute for Handicapped Research, and the Administration on Aging. Additional limited support from private foundations, United Way, and individuals has supplemented public funding.

RESEARCH AND EVALUATION

Design

To monitor the development of the CCODA program and to study its impact on service patterns, effectiveness and costs, On Lok has used three research approaches simultaneously. These are: (1) PROCESS ANALYSIS, that is, qualitative analysis to describe and interpret issues in program and systems development, including the use of the collected information related to program: (2) WITHIN GROUP STUDY, that is, ongoing collection of data related to

CCODA program participants, services and costs, with quantitative analysis of these data for use in program development, including the use of multiple regression techniques to assess for whom which services are most beneficial; and (3) COMPARATIVE STUDY, that is, quantitative analysis to assess relative program impacts, using a quasi-experimental (pre-multiple post matched-pair) design to compare the experiences of CCODA participants with similar elderly in the traditional long term care system.

The Process Analysis yields information about the program's development and operation; for example, referral sources and acceptance patterns. The Within Group Study includes data from all CCODA participants. The findings reported below result from data collected from all program participants from February 1979 through June 1982, a "CCODA Population" of 449 participants. The Comparative Study findings are based on data from 140 participants—a subset of 70 newly-admitted CCODA participants (called the "CCODA Group"), each matched with a non-CCODA counterpart (the "Comparison Group"). The Comparative Study's data cover a period from January 1980 through June 1982.

All participants in the CCODA program were assessed at regular intervals, usually every three months, by a multidisciplinary team of health professionals. That assessment covered health, functional and cognitive status. Services provided (inpatient and outpatient) by On Lok staff and by contracting specialists were recorded daily and tabulated monthly. An integrated cost accounting system was developed to track all costs and provide cost information by service category and participant. An on-line computerized information system was developed to manage, coordinate and integrate all of the information for the ongoing program. For those participating in the Comparative Study, health assessments covering medical, functional, cognitive status and expressed satisfaction were given at time of entry and at six month intervals thereafter. Service data were gathered using a health status questionnaire administered by research staff, and a cost instrument was used to track service costs. Up to two years of data (i.e., for assessments) were collected on Comparative Study participants. For participants in the program, data were gathered throughout their participation in the project.

A number of hypotheses were put forth for studying this project, the principal ones being:

- Days of institutionalization, both skilled and acute, would be lower for the CCODA Group while receipt of professional medical and therapeutic services would be higher.

* More health-related, social and rehabilitative services would be delivered to CCODA participants.
* Functional status of CCODA participants would improve over time.
* Long term care service costs would be lower for the CCODA Group.
* Costs would be distributed across a broader range of services and a lower proportion of cost would be accounted for by inpatient services.
* Public sector and total long term care costs would be lower for the CCODA Group.

The findings section that follows addresses these hypotheses using data from the ongoing program information system, comparative population data, and data from the Comparative Study. More detailed description of methods, measurement instruments, and study findings are available in other reports (Yordi & Waldman, 1982a, 1982b, 1983). The findings section which follows simply summarizes some of these results.

Findings

Inpatient days, both acute hospital and skilled nursing, were reduced as demonstrated from both program population data and data from the Comparative Study. In the twelve months of the calendar year 1982, On Lok served 326 participants for a total of 100,304 capitation days. For most of these days, program participants were able to receive the services they needed while remaining in the community. There were 1,319 acute hospital days during the year or 1.6% of total days; on a per capita basis, acute care usage for the CCODA population—which is predefined as a frail population— was only slightly higher, 4.8 days, than that of the entire 65 and older population in 1979, 4.2 days (DHHS, NCHS, 1981, p. 166). In addition, On Lok's participants used only 4,488 nursing home days or 4.5% of total capitation days for 1982.

The Comparative Study also demonstrated reduction in inpatient days. Days of acute care were 33% lower for the CCODA Group than the Comparison Group, 2% versus 3% of study days. In the Comparative Study, skilled nursing facility days were five times higher for the Comparison Group than the CCODA Group.

As might be expected, the reduction in institutional days was achieved through greater use of outpatient services. Almost all of On Lok's CCODA participants, for example, attended one of On Lok's day health centers at least once during each month with an average utilization around 13 days of attendance per month. Day health is not a universally available service so it is difficult to compare this utilization. The Comparative Study, however, does provide an estimate of the impacts of the CCODA program on health and community service utilization.

In the Comparative Study, the majority of the CCODA Group received services in an outpatient day health center, while the majority of the Comparison Group participants received services in their homes or in a skilled nursing facility. A significantly larger proportion of the CCODA Group than the Comparison Group received medical specialty services (namely, optometry, podiatry, dentistry and audiology), nursing, therapy, social services, meals, and transportation. Figure 2 compares the utilization by the two groups of outpatient and in-home services.

For the majority of the CCODA Population, use of outpatient services remained relatively stable over time; the exception was a gradual increase in personal care/home chore use—a 20% increase in the proportion of users over a two-year period as well as an increase in the volume of services (twice as high). One interesting finding from the CCODA project has been the extent of program control over inpatient services. In 1981 a new staff physician was hired, a HUD 202 facility was opened, and the service staff made a special effort to reduce inpatient utilization. Over the next year and a half, days in the acute hospital and days in skilled nursing facilities were cut in half. Nursing home days which were running above 9% were cut to a little more than 4% over a twelve-month period. Acute hospitalization which fluctuates considerably was averaging over 2% prior to 1981 and has since been brought down to an average of about 1% of capitation days.

The expectation for a frail older population is continued deterioration over time. With such an expectation, maintenance can be seen as a relative gain. Unfortunately, normative data is not available for assessing normal change in functional status for a long term care population. Comparative Study data thus provide an estimate of relative change in functional status. Over time, the majority of the

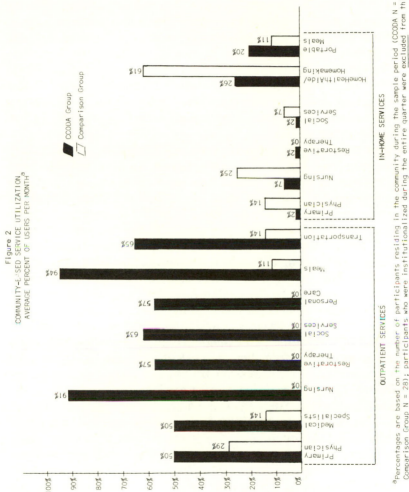

Figure 2

COMMUNITY-BASED SERVICE UTILIZATION
AVERAGE PERCENT OF USERS PER MONTH[a]

■ CCODA Group
□ Comparison Group

OUTPATIENT SERVICES

Primary Physician — 50%, 29%
Medical Specialists — 50%, 14%
Nursing — 91%, 0%
Restorative Therapy — 57%, 0%
Social Services — 63%, 0%
Personal Care — 57%, 0%
Meals — 94%, 11%
Transportation — 65%, 14%

IN-HOME SERVICES

Primary Physician — 2%, 14%
Nursing — 7%, 25%
Restorative Therapy — 2%, 0%
Social Services — 2%, 7%
Home Health Aide/Homemaking — 26%, 61%
Portable Meals — 20%, 11%

[a]Percentages are based on the number of participants residing in the community during the sample period (CCODA N = 48; Comparison Group N = 28); participants who were institutionalized during the entire quarter were excluded from this analysis.

159

CCODA Population improved or remained the same as measured by ten health and functional status indexes, e.g., cognition, activities of daily living (ADL), ability to compensate for illness. Relative to the Comparison Group, the CCODA Group experienced more improvement on all of the health and functional status indexes. The CCODA Group experienced greater improvement in their abilities to compensate for physical and mental limitations (such as impairments of their limbs or incontinence) than in the physical and mental conditions themselves.

The mortality rate for the CCODA Population was 157 per 1000. This is within the range cited for a nursing home population. In the Comparative Study, the mortality rate for the CCODA Group was comparable to that of the Comparison Group, 205 versus 224 per 1000 on an annual basis.

Over the three and one-half year study period, the average daily participant cost for the CCODA Population was $34.50 (1981 dollars) for all medical, social and supportive services provided either in the community or in inpatient facilities. It is difficult to compare absolute dollars, but this $34.50 for all services is at or below what Medicare would pay in California for just the room, board, and nursing services provided in the nursing home in San Francisco ($36.06 in 1981). In a typical month, the average daily participant cost ranged from as low as $1 to as high as $380, with the low end reflecting individuals whose health status required only very occasional monitoring and the high end reflecting those who used costly inpatient services. Variation in cost generally related to the level of care of the participant—the higher the impairment and dependency level, the higher the cost of care. As individual care needs intensified with increasing frailty, the average daily cost for individual CCODA participants rose gradually.

The Comparative Study showed that the average per capita cost of health care services for the Comparison Group was 26% higher than for the CCODA Group ($47.32 per day versus $37.50 per day). Even with adjustments for community living expenses such as housing, the total long term care cost (both public and private sectors) for the Comparison Group was still 12% higher than for the CCODA. While individual costs rose over time in both groups, the CCODA Group's cost increased at a slower rate. At the end of this first year of study, the cost difference between the two groups was $10.40; that difference had increased to $14.99 by the end of the second year.

Medically-oriented services (hospitals, nursing homes, physician services, etc.) dominate the traditional long term care system. However, nearly half (47%) of the CCODA's cost was spent on counseling, personal care, home chore, meals, recreation and transportation—social, supportive services. In the Comparative Study, inpatient cost (acute care and skilled nursing facility care) accounted for 25% of the CCODA Group's daily cost; whereas for the Comparison Group, 81% of the daily cost was incurred by institutional services.

In this demonstration project, the CCODA had single source funding by Medicare (with co-payments waived). But had the CCODA been under a traditional reimbursement mechanism, reimbursable services would only have amounted to 40% of the CCODA daily cost, or $13.80. That amount is substantially less than what Medicare ordinarily pays for such a frail population. (The frailty adjusted Average Area Per Capita Cost or "AAPCC" for Medicare is $584 per month or $19.20 per day.) Because information is lacking from other programs or sources that would cover the remaining 60% of the CCODA cost (Medicaid, Title XX, Title III of Older Americans Act, and out-of-pocket), fair comparison is impossible.

LESSONS LEARNED

All the numbers, findings and experiences of On Lok's last four years reveal a few important lessons.

The CCODA or consolidated model of care offers a number of advantages over traditional long term care and holds out a long sought hope—containing long term care costs while providing high quality care:

- Program participants have been able to live in their own homes or in community housing that allows maximum individual freedom and the opportunity for a higher quality of life.
- They receive more professional services (both in terms of quantity and range) and show more improvement in terms of functional independence than their counterparts.
- At the same time, On Lok's health care program costs were lower than those for a comparable sample of people in the neighboring community.

On Lok's multidisciplinary team, day health emphasis, control over resources and assumption of financial responsibility have been major factors in the CCODA's success:

- The use of the multidisciplinary team results not only in quality control, but also in a comprehensive, integrated response to the collection of problems each participant faces, rather than individual professional approaches to symptoms; continuity of care is assured as the various professionals who assess needs also work together to deliver the services.
- The day health center continues to prove itself an efficient way of delivering health services, providing the health professional more service time and making possible multiple services, group activities and more effective use of paraprofessionals; equally important is the stimulation participants provide for one another.
- Control over resources allows the team to prescribe and provide services according to need, without regard for payment mechanism. This flexibility also has meant cost savings, for On Lok could negotiate competitive fixed-rate contracts with participating consultants and facilities and provide appropriate lower cost "preventive" services, like transportation and supportive housing, to help reduce the use of such high cost services as hospitalization. Further, by avoiding the red tape associated with the traditional fee-for-service approach, On Lok could minimize its administrative costs.

Finally, none of these aspects of the CCODA were developed overnight. The development process was an ongoing one which started with On Lok's first day health center in the early 1970s. That process is the theme addressed by the discussion section below.

DISCUSSION: LONG TERM CARE PROGRAM LONGEVITY— ADAPTATION, SURVIVAL AND GROWTH

With the increasing interest in community-based long term care, the program-development life cycle of projects is a subject ripe for consideration. As community-based long term care projects go, On Lok at 12 years is an elder statesman. However, compared with the traditional long term care provider—the nursing home—On Lok is an early adolescent, full of promise and uncertainty. On Lok's ability to survive for more than a decade through adaptation to its environment and a succession of demonstration grants is somewhat unique. Its relative longevity is interesting from two standpoints: (1) why it has occurred—the anatomy of longevity; and (2) what its concomitant developments have been—the evolution of a program.

Anatomy of Longevity

On Lok has evolved over the years with energetic, stable leadership, unusual freedom and a strategy carefully tuned to: (1) the strengths and weaknesses of its community's service system; and (2) the funding opportunities available for the support of community-based long term care. In short, On Lok's long-term survival and growth can be attributed to five key factors: consistent leadership, freedom afforded by the organizational structure, the fit betwen the program and the community's service environment, incrementalism driven by vision, and a sense of timing and the political acumen to identify and seize opportunities.

First, as noted by Jessica Townsend in a recent study by the Institute of Medicine of the National Academy of Sciences (1982), On Lok's program has had consistent leadership, that is, virtually no turnover among its major designers and implementers. Despite dramatic changes in the program over time, two members of the initial group that launched On Lok in the 1960's still occupy the key board and executive staff positions. Similarly, the research unit, which has been an integral part of On Lok since the early days, has also enjoyed the same leadership from the beginning to the present.

The energy, dedication and individual qualifications shown by those guiding On Lok are not unique—in fact, they are common ingredients in community-based long term care programs. What is unique is the stability for more than a decade of a leadership *team.* Within the team, sparks may fly, styles may clash, but as a group they cover the bases and share a vision of community-based long term care. The continuity and diversity represented by this leadership undoubtedly has contributed to the program's momentum and strength over time. That continuity has enabled the program to learn from its mistakes and to refine its vision as more was learned.

Perhaps just as important in On Lok's progressive development as the continuity among On Lok's decisionmakers has been the freedom On Lok has enjoyed as a small, independent community-based organization. As a freestanding organization with no history, no bureaucracy, and no established reputation to protect, On Lok could experiment and take risks that would not have been possible had On Lok been part of a larger existing agency. The On Lok Board—with no status about which to be conscious—saw itself as the midwife for a new venture, not as the policeman to assure the program conformed to prescribed external standards. On Lok's size, newness and uniqueness also gave it the benefit of the doubt where external groups, such as state and local health departments, were concerned. On Lok, instead of having to fit the mold, was able to create its own forms and procedures and receive official support—rather than constraints—in the process.

On Lok's choice of program models—beginning with a day health center and moving gradually to a comprehensive, consolidated program—was shaped by the strength and weaknesses of its community service environment. On Lok exists in an inner city community whose residents are predominantly low income ethnic minorities—primarily Chinese, but also Italian and Filipino. The complex role of ethnicity—with multiple cultural values that have impeded as well as facilitated the development of On Lok—is beyond the scope of this paper. However, two characteristics of On Lok's geographically defined community have been of clear importance to program success: its sense of neighborhood identity and the presence of substantial informal supports for its older residents. On Lok taps that community to keep its service quality high—its three centers' doors are always open, and the constant flow of school groups, family members, associations and media representatives through the centers places the service program under continuous scrutiny.

Broad community support was not immediate, nor did it have to be, given the nature and small scale of On Lok's original project. Yet, after six years, the program had gained sufficient acceptance and visibility that it could embark upon and succeed in two "impossible" ventures. On the one hand, it was able to build in the heart of the high-rent district, a six-story, 54-unit housing facility for the area's frail elderly, complete with a day health center on its ground floor. On another front, On Lok increased its program size from 80 to 300 and radically altered the health care delivery system for those served, by changing from only a day health program into a comprehensive health care system.

From the outset, On Lok's goal has been the same: to provide an environment and the supportive services to enable the elderly to remain in their own community so long as it is medically, socially and economically feasible. It has proceeded *incrementally* towards this vision, however, One by one, small steps have been taken to implement the grand plan. The small steps have ensured that the program is built on a firm base of community support and that its managerial and service staff capabilities are equal to the tasks. Thus, although the entire new CCODA system was operational within one year after its demonstration phase began, this demonstration began with a great deal already in place: two day centers, six years operational experience and community acceptance. Even so, new contractual relationships had to be established (vendors chosen, rates negotiated), the cooperation of community professionals (especially private physicians) had to be enlisted and participants recruited. So, even with On Lok's base, it took *three years* for the CCODA program to reach full census.

On Lok's small-step approach has meant flexibility—On Lok had many options to pursue, many pieces to offer funders. Accordingly, On Lok's sustained growth is in no small way due to its capacity to read the political winds and play the right cards. This has not been a case of changing the program to accommodate changes in administration. Rather it has been a matter of phasing in the components at the appropriate time. A closer look at the manner in which the On Lok program has evolved makes this process clear.

The Evolution of a Program

When On Lok began, its immediate environment included no traditional long term care providers. Indeed, the presenting problem was the absence of long term care facilities in the community. The community itself offered only limited, discrete services—some home health care, homemaker chore services, medical services through private physicians and acute care hospitals.

On Lok's founders explored the "obvious" solution of building a nursing home in the area and quickly dismissed that alternative as neither feasible nor desirable given the high cost of San Francisco real estate and the difficulties seen in nursing home care. Instead they decided to pursue the development of a protective housing facility and a system of outpatient services, modeled after the day centers in England (Cosin, 1970, 1971). Significantly, the British day hospital model was considered as promising not just by the few who were seeking a solution for the frail elderly in Chinatown-

North Beach, but also by the Administration on Aging (AoA). Seizing the opportunity, On Lok applied for funds from AoA to begin implementing its grand plan of a continuum of care.

To the surprise of many, On Lok was included with Burke Rehabilitation Center, Levindale Geriatric Center, and Montefiori as one of the four projects throughout the nation awarded funds to plan, develop and evaluate a day center program for the elderly. With renovation, an old nightclub was transformed into a storefront day center, licensed as an outpatient community clinic and opened to participants in March 1973. The early emphasis of the program was on social support: meals, recreational activities, personal care and social services. On Lok continued to develop and evolve, primarily in response to participant needs but also in part to reimbursement contingencies.

Almost immediately, On Lok secured the interest of the State of California. On Lok planners, aware that demonstration funds could not provide the long-term, stable support needed by the project, opened discussions with the California State Department of Health regarding Medicaid reimbursement for the day center program. After 1-1/2 years of negotiations, On Lok began its first Medicaid demonstration in December of 1974.

The Medicaid demonstration had a pronounced impact on the development of On Lok's day center program. With emphasis focused on the medical services delivered through the program, medical and personal care needs of the average participant increased. Medicaid reimbursement required more extensive and detailed recordkeeping than did the AoA demonstration project, and since health recording systems for a day center service program did not exist, On Lok had to develop the system. Medicaid reimbursement also forced out participants with only social supportive needs. Many of these participants returned to the community and, without social support, again developed the same medical problems that brought them to On Lok's day health center the first time.

In the summer of 1975, On Lok faced a practical problem—survival. Its AoA day center demonstration was over, and Medicaid reimbursement for On Lok's day center services was not enough to sustain the On Lok program. Some participants, for example, were not Medicaid eligible and thus were not covered; some needed services—for example, chore service, portable meals, home health—which could no longer be provided under the Medicaid demonstration.

Accordingly, On Lok submitted a new application to AoA—this time, for a Model Project on Aging grant to develop and refine its day health center, and with it as a base, establish an outpatient continuum of care. In moving towards a continuum of care, the Model Project on Aging Grant called for: (1) the development of a second day center designed for the elderly without medical problems but with psycho-social needs which could be met through a social health maintenance program; (2) in-home services including portable meals, chore services, and home health care as an adjunct to the day center program; and (3) work on the housing problems of On Lok's elderly participants.

Through a series of extensions, On Lok's Model Project on Aging grant lasted three years and seven months until late 1978. During that period, while On Lok continually battled for financial support, the program evolved from a day center to an outpatient continuum of care offering health and health-related services to the functionally dependent adult. One of the most remarkable accomplishments was the development of "On Lok House," a congregate housing facility combining housing separate from, but together with, a full range of health services. By 1978, a site had been purchased, plans developed, HUD 202 funds with Section 8 waivers secured, and construction begun. Further, during the Model Project On Lok at last secured permanency for a portion of its program: through AB 1611 passed in 1977, day health became a regular Medicaid benefit.

Although the expanded outpatient program was an improvement, it still was not enough. The private physician still had ultimate control over the participant's medical care. In many instances, the private physician, not being involved with the multidisciplinary team, would work at odds with a participant's plan of care. In addition, without inpatient services, the system of long term health care was incomplete. Once a participant was institutionalized, the On Lok program had limited resources for returning that person to the community. Thus, On Lok learned that nursing homes, hospitals and medical care all had to be integrated with outpatient therapeutic, social and supportive services into a single health care system.

As a result, On Lok sought and won funding in October 1978 from the Office of Human Development Services for a four-year effort to plan, develop and study the CCODA—an extension of the continuum to include *all* health and health-related services to the "long term care" elderly. Within only four months, HCFA had granted the necessary waivers to implement the service program, a process undoubtedly hastened by On Lok's research and development funding from a third party.

The CCODA demonstration, Phase I, was to end in February 1983. Once again, On Lok battled to save its successful demonstration from extinction. The CCODA experience had shown the program to be good both for those it served and for those who paid for it. Yet there still were problems. Although cost-effective, the CCODA did not have a realistic funding base, nor did it have permanence. To move from its Medicare-only demonstration status, On Lok proposed to spread cost responsibility (Medicare, Medicaid and private copayments) and to put On Lok at financial risk. When selling this phase to HCFA proved futile, On Lok had to take extraordinary, unprecedented action. On Lok took its arguments directly to Congress, with the result that Section 603(c) of the Conference Report on the Social Security Amendments of 1983 provides the Secretary shall approve "the risk-sharing application of On Lok Senior Health Services for [Medicare and Medicaid] waivers . . . in order to carry out a [36-month] demonstration project for capitated reimbursement for comprehensive long term care services . . ." At this writing, On Lok is about to embark on its fifth major demonstration project. Even with legislated "approval," administrative requirements for new Medicare and Medicaid waivers must be negotiated with HCFA.

After 12 years of growth and success, only a portion of On Lok's community-based program is permanently secure—the day health package for Medicaid-eligible participants. The question remains as to whether On Lok's new, congressionally-mandated demonstration will lead, at last, to permanent funding for the entire program and others like it as with day health services.

CONCLUSION

On Lok has successfully met the objectives of its various demonstrations and has used these mechanisms to build its program over the years. It has even succeeded in gaining state legislation for the permanent reimbursement of some of its components (i.e., Medicaid reimbursement for day health) and obtaining national legislation to extend its progress toward permanent status for the entire program. Despite its successes, it still shares common problems with other community-based long term care demonstrations.

The reality of a demonstration service program is a continual battle for financial support, a battle which draws energy away from the program's stated objectives. Many governmental agencies will sponsor demonstrations, but for a limited period of time only, usually three years or less. The idea usually is to develop a new system, assess it and then stop it, regardless of its impacts.

Such a demonstration model is not realistic. First, a new service program cannot simply be "turned on" and "turned off," but must develop and evolve. New service programs need to develop procedures, establish a census, make their mistakes and learn; all these activities take time. Usually by the end of a time-limited demonstration, a program is only then beginning to function in a somewhat effective manner. With the policy of time-limited demonstrations and a reluctance of agencies to re-fund the same project, demonstration programs usually must either close down or change. As a result, any progress made through the demonstration is usually lost.

Not every successful demonstration has the political capability to change health care policy. Even those that do orient themselves to policy change cannot immediately effect the policy change. On Lok's original 1972-75 research and demonstration project established a day health center, yet it took three years more for the refinement of the program and passage of state legislation for its ongoing support.

Program survival beyond a promising infancy should not depend on the special situations On Lok has been able to create for itself. In contrast to demonstration efforts, established traditional health services have secure reimbursement. It is time to recognize that successful community-based long term care demonstrations need secure reimbursement too, if they are to play a serious role in solving this country's long term care crisis.

REFERENCES

Cosin, L. Z. Testimony before the Subcommittee on Long Term Care of Senate Special Committee on Aging. *Congressional Record,* December 1970, June 1971.

Kalish, R., Lurie, E., Wexler, R., & Zawadski, R. *On Lok Senior Health Services: Evaluation of a success.* San Francisco: On Lok Senior Health Services, 1975.

RTZ Associates. *Adult day health services: Its impacts on the frail elderly and the quality and cost of long term care* (5 reports). Sacramento: California State Department of Health Publications, May 1977.

Townsend, Jessica. On Lok Senior Health Services (Case report). In Institute of Medicine, Committee on Services Integration. *Health services Integration: Lessons for the 1980s* (Vol. 3 of final report, Publication No. (10M) 82-03C). Washington, DC: National Academy Press, 1982.

U.S. Congress, House. *Conference report to Social Security Amendments of 1983* (H.R. Report No. 98-47). Report to accompany H.R. 1900, 98th Congress, 1st Session, March 24, 1983.

U.S. Department of Health and Human Services, National Center for Health Statistics. *Health , United States, 1981* (DHHS Publication No. (PHS) 82-1232). Washington, DC: U.S. Government Printing Office, 1981.

Von Behren, R. *On Lok Senior Health Services adult day health care—From pilot project to permanent program* (Final report). Sacramento: California State Department of Health Publications, July 1979.

Yordi, C. L., & Waldman, J. *A comparative study of the traditional long term care system and a consolidated model of long term care.* Unpublished manuscript, 1983. (Available from On Lok Senior Health Services, 1455 Bush Street, San Francisco, CA 94109).

Yordi, C. L., & Waldman, J. *A comparative study on the quality and cost of long term care for the frail elderly: The research design and sampling methodology* (Technical Report No. 306). San Francisco: On Lok Senior Health Services, September 1982.

Yordi, C. L., & Waldman, J. *Assessing the relative impacts of a coordinated system of long term care: A conceptual model, assessment protocols and data collection procedures* (Technical Report No. 307). San Francisco: On Lok Senior Health Services, September 1982.

Zawadski, R. T. *On Lok Senior Health Services: Toward a continuum of care.* San Francisco: On Lok Senior Health Services, 1979.

Chapter 9

Triage:
A Long Term Care Study

Joan L. Quinn, MSN
Joseph H. Hodgson, MSW

OVERVIEW

Triage was developed as a model project for the coordinated delivery of medical and social services to the elderly. Unlike the traditional system where the services provided to an individual depend
upon what is available and reimbursable, Triage organized services
around the needs of the client, stimulated the development of new
services where needed ones were not available, and assured that all
needed services were adequately monitored and reimbursed. Its purpose was to test the effectiveness and to measure the costs of this
system of delivering care to the elderly.

Two underlying principles guided the operation of the Triage program:

- Intervention should foster maximum independence and functioning ability; and,
- Intervention should provide health care services which were
most appropriate and sensitive to the individual client's needs.

When Triage became operational on February 1, 1974, it resem-
bled a health maintenance organization without walls, focused on

Joan L. Quinn is former Executive Director of Triage, Inc., and President, Connecticut
Community Care, Inc. Bristol, Connecticut. Joseph H. Hodgson is former Assistant Direc-
tor/Community Relations of Triage, Inc., and Consultant, Joseph H. Hodgson and
Associates, West Simsbury, Connecticut.

Questions may be directed to Joan L. Quinn, MSN, Executive Director, Triage, Inc.;
President, Connecticut Community Care, Inc.; 719 Middle Street, Bristol, CT 06010.

171

meeting the multiple needs of the older adult. Triage was a free-standing agency which assumed an advocacy, coordination and brokerage role for both the elderly and service providers themselves. The Triage project represented the first time that a full spectrum of medical and non-medical services for older people were incorporated under a unified prescriptive mechanism with a single funding source.

The single reimbursement system proved to be a most efficient mechanism for controlling costs, coordinating services and assuring quality of care. Thus, the Triage model proved to be an important factor in the evolution of future long term care models around the country, despite the fact that the Triage organization itself was dissolved with the loss of federal funding.

PROJECT ORIGIN AND OBJECTIVES

The Triage project, a cooperative venture between the state and federal governments, had as its stimulus the 1971 White House Conference on Aging which had highlighted the deficiencies of the existing fragmented, poorly-funded "non-system" of care. A determination to try to create in Connecticut a comprehensive, cost-effective long term care system resulted in the beginning of the project.

Project Triage began in February 1974 with state funding and a start-up grant from the federal Administration on Aging (Older Americans Act, Title IIIA Model Project of National Scope Grant). Triage's prime objectives were to increase the range and availability of services and to coordinate service delivery within a seven-town region in central Connecticut (Berlin, Bristol, Burlington, New Britain, Plainville, Plymouth, and Southington). The central Connecticut region was typical of the rest of the state in the proportion of the elderly among the total population, with similar ethnicity, urban-rural mix, and general socio-economic characteristics. Thus, it was deemed a suitable microcosm in which to test the Triage model.

The governing body of Project Triage was Triage, Inc., a private, voluntary nonprofit organization that was a consortium of board members from provider agencies and elderly consumers representative of the seven towns served by the project. The board of directors was composed of persons nominated by the area's hospitals and community health agencies plus a consumer representative from each town.

Joint state-federal efforts resulted in two subsequent phases of Triage. Between April 1, 1976 and March 31, 1979, federal funding was provided under a research grant to the Connecticut State Department on Aging from the National Center for Health Services Research, Public Health Service, U.S. Department of Health, Education and Welfare. The State Department on Aging in turn contracted with Triage, Inc. for operations and with the University of Connecticut Health Center for evaluation. For the period from April 1, 1979 through September 30, 1981, the Health Care Financing Administration, U.S. Department of Health and Human Services granted Triage continued funding for Phase II of project operations and evaluation.

At the outset of the demonstration project, five primary objectives were established for Triage. They were to:

1. provide a single entry mechanism to coordinate delivery of institutional, ambulatory and in-home services on behalf of the elderly client;
2. develop necessary preventive and supportive services;
3. develop an integrated service delivery system at the local level;
4. obtain public and private financial support for the full spectrum of services;
5. demonstrate the cost-effectiveness of coordinated care, including:
   a. care to compensate for disability and support independent living at home;
   b. care prescribed appropriate to need rather than according to third-party payor service restrictions.

PROJECT CHARACTERISTICS

Population Served

During the seven and one-half years of Triage operations, a total of 2,628 people were enrolled in the program. A maximum of 1,750 were served at any one time during Triage I (prior to April 1979), but this number was reduced to 1,500 during Triage II. In addition, during most of the Triage program period, 2,100 persons were on a waiting list as enrollment was limited because of staff size and grant limitations.

An eligible person became a Triage client by referral, most frequently by individual elderly applicants themselves, but also by families, friends or neighbors, visiting nurses, hospital discharge planners, physicians, and social workers. Some potential clients wanted to use the service for its insurance value, i.e., services reimbursed by the Triage program. Most often, program enrollment was sought because the family and/or the service provider could no longer cope with the problems of the older person or because the community was concerned about protecting the older person. Elderly people often referred themselves to Triage for security reasons. Many clients took the position that while they did not need help at the time of referral, they might need it in the future. Clients on the Triage waiting list often stated that it was comforting to be on the waiting list because they would be known to the program if they "got into trouble."

During Phase I of the project, the only requirements for becoming a client were age (60 years old), Medicare eligibility, and residence in the seven-town Triage area. However, a major change occurred in the criteria for enrollment under Triage II. Because of reduced resources and grant limitations as to the number to be served (1500), staff determined that only those who were at high risk of institutionalization and who might benefit most from the Triage intervention were accepted as new clients. Criteria for being considered "high risk" included the need for Triage assessment coordination, and monitoring of medical and social services, and the existence of a fragil or unstable informal support system. As a result, the new enrollees of Triage II had more complicated health problems and poorer functional status. They were generally less able to obtain needed care from family and friends than those clients who were enrolled during Triage I. Under Triage II, 495 persons were enrolled using the high risk eligibility criteria. An additional 1,402 of those already enrolled in Triage I continued as clients during Triage II.

The Triage population served consisted of a frail elderly group, predominantly widowed females, who lived alone with less than adequate financial resources and limited educational attainment. Only 14% of the Triage population had incomes of over $6,000 per year ($500 per month). More than half (58%) of the Triage population were over 75 years old at the initial assessment, compared to Connecticut's aging population over 75 (28%) and the nation's (27%). At the end of the project's first grant period, 60.3% of the program's active client population were over 75. These age characteristics become important when one considers that people over 75 are five times as likely to be institutionalized as those under 75.

Service Program

The primary components of the Triage model were assessment of health and social needs; coordination of care; monitoring of services and client status; and client and family education about the health care system. The result was an individualized plan of care for each client that could be modified to meet changing health care needs.

Lack of knowledge or confusion about service type, service availability and reimbursement was expressed by the majority of referred individuals. For many people, the aging process itself was not understood, and therefore understanding their health condition was seen as problematic.

Assessment. Assessment consisted of a modified physical examination and an extensive health interview. A nurse-clinician or a nurse-clinician/social service coordinator team completed this comprehensive assessment during a home visit. The interview included a complete health history (i.e., physical and mental problems of an acute and chronic nature, prescription and non-prescription drugs taken) and information on the client's functional status, social background, nutrition, physical environment, and living expenditures. Functional status was assessed using three standardized instruments:

- the Activities of Daily Living (ADL), which measures the ability to perform the most basic functions such as bathing, dressing, eating and toileting (Katz, Ford, Moskowitz, Jackson, & Jaffee, 1963);
- the Instrumental Activities of Daily Living (IADL), which measures the ability to perform daily household and functional tasks, such as shopping, telephoning, cooking, taking medication, and handling money (Lawton & Brody, 1969); and,
- the Mental Status Questionnaire (MSQ), which measures the client's cognitive functioning (Kahn, Goldfarb, Pollack, & Gerber, 1960).

The assessment incorporated the person's value system by bringing functional status and health status variables together from both an objective and self-reporting viewpoint. The assessment tool itself provided the basis for the problem-oriented client record (Weed, 1971), which was developed at the completion of the initial assessment.

Available services, the plan of care and service coordination. The scope of potential services was extensive. Home health aide, homemaker service, nursing, physician visits, psychological counseling, transportation, home-delivered meals, chore service, companion service, hospital care, nursing home care, dental care, financial counseling, pharmaceuticals, medical supplies and equipment, physical therapy, audiology, podiatry, and optometry were among the services available. Based on the total assessment and the resultant client problem list, a plan of care appropriate to meeting each client's needs was developed. Working with the client and his or her family, the Triage team began to select the available services which were appropriate and the providers who should be asked to deliver the services.

To initiate a service, a member of the Triage team telephoned a provider and established the kind and amount of services to be rendered, date for services to begin, and a re-evaluation date for service continuation. This verbal arrangement was confirmed through a written service order, authorizing payment for services rendered. Bills were sent directly to Triage, not the client, for reimbursement processing.

After the delivery of services commenced, the Triage team maintained continual contact with the client to assure that the quantity and quality of the services were meeting his or her current needs. Changes in the quantity and mix of services occurred as needs changed. Progress notes were made in the client's record on the basis of telephone calls and/or home visits. The team also consulted frequently with the service providers. Providers were required to submit reports which detailed the client's status, the services rendered, and the instructions given by the provider to the client.

Funding and Financing Mechanism

Beginning in August 1975, comprehensive waivers for the use of Medicare Trust Funds were awarded in support of Project Triage by the Secretary of the Department of Health, Education and Welfare under the authority granted through Section 222 of P.L. 92-603 (the Social Security Amendments of 1972). Waivers granted to the project were as follows:

- *Waiver of duration, amount and scope of services* - allowing Triage to authorize payment for many ancillary and supportive services not traditionally covered by Medicare, such as pharmaceuticals, dental care, mental health services, homemaker services, glasses, and hearing aids.
- *Waiver of specific Medicare requirements* - allowing Triage to forego deductibles and coinsurance, as well as several restrictions on home health care. For example, these waivers lifted the restrictions placed upon an older adult's ability to receive health care by eliminating the physician plan of care, the need for skilled nursing, and the Medicare requirement that the individual be "home-bound."

The federal fiscal intermediary (the agency which determines the reasonable costs of services and reimburses the providers) for Project Triage was the Office of Direct Reimbursement (ODR) of the Health Care Financing Administration (HCFA). Triage was responsible for verifying client eligibility and authorizing payment of providers by ODR. All bills for prescribed services were directed to the Triage office for review and approval and then forwarded to ODR, which issued payment to the provider. Reimbursement was limited to those services specifically authorized in writing by the Triage clinical teams.

While most service costs continued to be reimbursed from Medicare Trust Funds, a new financial participation policy was adopted at the inception of Triage II to encourage cost consciousness on the part of the client. Clients were asked for contributions to help defray the costs for those waivered services which would otherwise have to be self-paid in their entirety. The amounts requested took into account individual income, the personal value to the client of the waivered service or set of services, and the cost of the service. The suggested copayments ranged from 3% to 15% of the cost of the waivered services. A client was able, however, to choose an amount outside of this range. Furthermore, although financial participation was encouraged it was not a prerequisite for program eligibility.

During the 1979-1981 grant period, Triage clients contributed a total of $393,985—10% of the cost of the waivered services. All contributions were returned to the Medicare Trust Funds. The contributions themselves were significant because they represented a high rate of participation in cost-sharing among the client population. This population had not been expected to contribute to the cost of care under the initial grant.

RESEARCH AND EVALUATION

To determine the impact of Triage on functional status, utilization and costs, and to offer policymakers objective information crucial for evaluating options for oganizing and financing long term care, Triage's research endeavors were focused on three groups: (1) the total Triage population enrolled since the beginning of the program (5-1/2 years); (2) the Triage high risk group enrolled in Triage II (1979-1981); and (3) an experimental and comparison group. Client functional status, client service utilization and costs, and the probability of service utilization as a function of time were studied in each group. Due to space limitations, only the results from the experimental-comparison group analyses are presented and over-time data are not considered.

Research Design

The experimental group consisted of all Triage clients assessed from August 1, 1976 through January 31, 1977 ($n = 289$). The comparison group was constructed from a population of older persons living in a demographically similar area in another part of the state ($n = 175$). The groups were matched on some salient sociodemographic characteristics and on initial scores on the Activities of Daily Living and the Instrumental Activities of Daily Living measures.

Each individual was given an initial assessment followed by periodic reassessments every six months. Service utilization data for the experimental group were obtained from one source, Project Triage billing records. Data for the comparison group had to be compiled from four different sources: (1) participant diaries, (2) provider records, (3) Medicare records, and (4) Medicaid reports.

The approach used, therefore, focused on the total estimated costs of some specific health care services affected by the Triage program, including nursing home costs and costs of health support and social services delivered in the home by formal providers. While Triage had little control over client utilization and costs of physician and hospital services, these costs were also compared for the two study groups because Medicare waivers of coinsurance and deductibles were granted under the Triage program for these services.

Two difficult methodological problems were encountered. First, the experimental and comparison group members differed in their functional status characteristics. Second, the health resources available in the two areas differed.

The first problem was partially resolved by matching the groups as closely as possible on several salient variables. However, the proportion of members age 75 and over at initial assessment was higher in the experimental group (59%) than in the comparison group (48%), and more of the experimental group scored less than the maximum of ten on the Mental Status Questionnaire (MSQ) (35%, as opposed to 18% in the comparison group).

The second problem was impossible to overcome fully. While the central cities of the Triage service area (New Britian and Bristol) share many socioeconomic characteristics with the central city of the comparison group area (Norwich), the central Connecticut area of Triage is much closer to the Hartford or Capitol Region and a greater supply of hospital beds, nursing home beds, and physicians. Essential home care elements such as homemaker, chore and companion services were also underdeveloped or almost nonexistent in the comparison group area, as they were in the Triage area prior to the resource development efforts undertaken during the first phase of the project.

Findings

Impact on functional status. Changes in functional status between initial assessment and last reassessment were measured for the Triage demonstration (experimental) group (289) and the matched non-Triage comparison group. (The last reassessment occurred anywhere from six months to five years after the initial assessment.) Measures of change in functional status included proportion of group with improved, maintained and declined functional status, and median change in functional status.

High statistical variability in the study populations, combined with small sample size and relatively insensitive measures of functional status, may have obscured some of the results. Some of the specific statistical tests showed a positive impact of Triage intervention; others did not. However, considering results from all of the tests, the Triage experimental group appears to have experienced a pattern of improved functional status between initial assessment and last reassessment, compared to the non-Triage comparison group (see Table 1).

Impact on utilization and costs. The principal findings of the util-

Table 1

CHANGES IN FUNCTIONAL STATUS
BETWEEN INITIAL ASSESSMENT AND LAST REASSESSMENT BY GROUP

	Percent Improving	Percent Declining	Change In Median Score[a]
ADL			
Experimental	9	33	-.11
Comparison	6	30	-.09
IADL			
Experimental	17	61	-.64
Comparison	15	63	-.68
MSQ			
Experimental	14	31	-.12
Comparison	6	24	-.14

[a]On the ADL, scores can range from 0 (totally dependent) to 7 (Independent); on the IADL, from 0 (totally dependent) to 8 (Independent); and on the MSQ, from 0 (disoriented) to 10 (full cognitive abilities).

ization and cost comparisons were that the Triage experimental group:

- used less than half the nursing home days of the comparison group;
- had approximately the same total cost for nursing home and home health services as the comparison group; and
- had higher hospital and physician costs than the comparison group; however, the comparison group area was characterized by fewer medical resources and a pattern of lower hospital utilization.

Utilization of medical and social services by the Triage experimental group and the comparison group was examined from three perspectives: the proportion of clients using a particular service, the mean units per client, and the mean units per user. As shown in Table 2, the Triage experimental group clients were only half as likely as those in the comparison group to enter a nursing home. Triage was successful in helping many clients who entered nursing homes return home when their functioning status and/or family support situation improved. The average number of days used per Triage experimental group member was about half that found for

Table 2
UTILIZATION OF SERVICES PER SIX-MONTH PERIOD:
EXPERIMENTAL AND COMPARISON GROUPS

Proportion Using Services	Experimental	Comparison
Skilled Nursing Facility	0.04	0.09
Visiting Nurse	0.34	0.06
Therapy	0.02	0.00
Home Health Aide	0.16	0.03
Homemaker	0.18	0.00
Chore	0.13	0.00
Companion	0.04	0.00

Mean Units Per Client	Experimental	Comparison
Skilled Nursing Facility	4.32	9.32
Visiting Nurse	2.06	0.24
Therapy	0.15	0.00
Home Health Aide	10.93	0.67
Homemaker	8.44	0.00
Chore	3.14	0.00
Companion	3.14	0.00

Mean Units Per User[a]	Experimental	Comparison
Skilled Nursing Facility	66.47	95.14
Visiting Nurse	6.44	3.25
Therapy	5.57	0.00
Home Health Aide	57.37	8.71
Homemaker	44.79	0.00
Chore	22.81	0.00
Companion	102.46	0.00

Note. The statistics in this table are median estimates of means developed from the median polish technique (Tukey, 1977) described in Volume II of the Triage II Final Report. This technique reduces the effects of statistical outliers on estimates of the mean. Because the statistics shown are estimates of means rather than computed sample means, products of units per user and the proportions using services may not equal units per client.

[a]Units of measure are days for skilled nursing facility; visits for visiting nurse and therapy; and hours for home health aide, homemaker, chore, and companion.

the comparison group, and the number of mean days per user was about 30% less for the Triage experimental group than for the comparison group (66 days versus 95 days).

Triage clients' lower nursing home utilization reflected a substitution of home health and social services for nursing home care. For each of the home health and social services, utilization by Triage clients far exceeded the comparison group's. The only home health services used at all by the comparison group—visiting nurse and home health aide—are traditionally covered by Medicare. Even for those services, however, the comparison group's utilization was significantly lower.

Nursing home costs were substantially lower for the Triage experimental group than for the comparison group while the reverse was true for home care costs (see Table 3). The total cost of nursing

Table 3

ESTIMATED COST PER PERSON PER SIX-MONTH PERIOD:
EXPERIMENTAL AND COMPARISON GROUPS

	Cost Per Unit (Estimated 1981 Prices)	Experimental Group	Comparison Group
Skilled Nursing Facility	$45	$194.34	$419.32
Visiting Nurse	28	57.72	6.60
Therapy	25	3.80	0.00
Home Health Aide	9	98.40	5.99
Homemaker	8	67.51	0.00
Chore	4	12.55	0.00
Companion	4	12.57	0.00
Total SNF and Home Health Care		$446.89	$431.91
Hospital (unadjusted)	$250	$992.50	$423.28
Physician (unadjusted)	30	178.14	94.33
Total Health (unadjusted)		$1,547.53	$949.52
Hospital (adjusted)	$250	992.50	671.75
Physician (adjusted	30	178.14	235.82
Total Health (adjusted)		$1,547.53	$1,339.48

home and home health care for the Triage experimental group was about 3% higher than for the comparison group. For the comparison group, the supply of home care services not traditionally covered by Medicare, such as chore and companion, was virtually nonexistent. Triage, on the other hand, increased its area's supply of home care services considerably.

Hospital and physician costs were higher for the Triage experimental than for the comparison group. Unlike home health care, which was authorized by the Triage professional team, physician and hospital services were provided by and/or under the direction of physicians. That is, Triage had little impact on their use other than in requesting initial physician visits.

Because both the comparison and the Triage experimental group were older and were in poorer health than the overall Medicare population, their hospital and physician costs could reasonably be expected to be higher than those of the Medicare population as a whole, by a factor of 1.25 to 2.0. Yet the comparison group's costs were lower: annual hospital costs ($847) were only 65% of the national average ($1,300), and physician costs ($189) were only 34% of the national average ($560) (Health Care Financing Administration, 1982). To reflect more normal or expected utilization patterns, the comparison group hospital and physician cost data were adjusted (by multiplying the hospital cost estimate by 1/.63, and the physician cost by 1/.40). These correction factors took into account both regional differences in utilization patterns (Connecticut Statewide Health Coordinating Council, 1979) and the difference between the comparison group expenditures and the HCFA national estimates.

After these adjustments in hospital and physician costs, the estimate of total health costs for the comparison group was a figure much closer to, but still less than, the figure for the experimental group ($1,339 versus $1,548). Hidden costs in the Medicare program such as fiscal intermediary expenditure were not considered in this comparison.

LESSONS LEARNED

The efficient and compassionate delivery of medical and social services requires the effective allocation of available resources. Historically, this resource allocation has been approached from two ostensibly different positions. On the one hand, a consumer-oriented, advocacy stance has focused discussions of resource allocation upon service development (options) and service procurement (access). On the other hand, the insurance or transfer benefit position has focused resource allocation discussion upon issues of financial risk and cash flow (reimbursement).

At the center of the long term care dilemma is the fragmentation between health care consumers, providers of service and public/private reimbursement groups. This fragmentation prohibits the collaborative application of available resources and results in costly health care system inefficiencies.

The Triage experience yielded important lessons germane to broad policy and program operational issues.

- Fit the reimbursement system to people's needs. The Medicare and Medicaid programs, as presently constructed, provide benefits for a restricted set of health care services, encouraging inpatient care over home health care. For many, this approach has resulted in unnecessary institutionalization, leading to deterioration in both health and functional status and higher costs. Benefits should be broadened to include expanded home care services, particularly those of a social nature (i.e., homemaker, chore, and companion).
- Cost sharing can be an effective cost containment tool. During Triage II, voluntary cost sharing was introduced. Accepted by most clients, it increased client sensitivity to the issue of cost versus need and heightened client interest in monitoring service quality and preventing provider abuses. The elimination of cost sharing for hospital and physician care, which occurred under Triage, is not an *essential* component of a Triage-type program; removing many Medicare restrictions on hospital and physician services undoubtedly contributed to increased utilization of those services.
- Cost sharing can be incorporated into health benefit programs for the elderly; however, its structure should either encourage home health care over institutional care or be neutral between the two. The current bias toward institutional care both adds to cost and leads to inappropriate use.
- An assessment, coordination and monitoring program should be independent of provision of services. An organization which has a financial interest in providing services may not be best suited for monitoring services. It may not be able to remain un-

biased between its own and others' services. Regardless of whether the organization is voluntary or for profit, incentives to expand the provision of services will tend to inhibit the performance of its monitoring function.

- The comprehensive assessment procedure is an important decision making vehicle for older people. This decision making process allows reallocation of personal resources and enables children to invest in the welfare of their older family member in a system that works for the entire family constellation. Through this cooperative venture, dysfunctioning family units can be kept at a minimum.

- Counseling and support services provided to the client and family members help them adjust to the needs of the long term care consumer. A sense of confusion, despair, and even crisis can be alleviated by counseling and information on specific problems and services available from specific providers.

- Current policy developments in long term care convey the message that the only time people are entitled to service is when they are in crisis, whether it be the client or a family member. The focus of long term care policy should be on preventing the crisis from occurring in the first place.

- A Triage type of health care delivery system requires a continuous review of the functions of client assessment, coordination and monitoring of services to prevent system rigidity and to maintain a climate favorable to dynamic organization initiatives. A new system such as Triage requires a different interdisciplinary health professional and a different viewpoint on caring for and bringing services to older people.

DISCUSSION: LIFE AFTER DEMONSTRATION

The Triage model constituted an experiment in changing the service delivery mechanism for long term care. Other programs had tested the effectiveness of discrete, innovative long term care services and showed that the problems of health care delivery for the elderly could not be "fixed" simply by expanding the number of reimbursable services under Medicare or Medicaid to include one or two unique services. What was needed instead was a system change, an integration of medical and non-medical service delivery.

The conclusion of the seven-year demonstration period generated a formidable predicament for both Triage and the federal government. While the project represented one of the most comprehensive undertakings in long term care research, it also represented the first time that a major demonstration was to be terminated. The federal officials overseeing the Triage project appeared to lack any substantive understanding of the impact of termination upon the client population. There was no federal willingness to negotiate the development of an ongoing client assistance mechanism which could: (1) assure that termination would occur in a reasoned and careful manner; and (2) provide continued support to Triage clients and their families. The burden of actual termination thus fell upon Triage staff, who were left with less than 60 working days in which to terminate over 1,000 clients living in the community who were dependent upon Triage case management and health care services.

Triage had experienced almost yearly threats to its continued existence, having been funded over its seven years with varying proportions of federal and state monies. Crises occurred at fiscal year ends—June 30 (state) or September 30 (federal)—giving Triage administrative staff few months of the year free from negotiation for continued funding. Fortunately, even with continued uncertainty, Triage had minimal staff turnover. This has not held true for other programs with similar fiscal difficulties. In all, the Triage project operated in an uneasy atmosphere, requiring tremendous motivational support among all staff for one another and placing unique and taxing demands upon the executive director.

While administrative staff negotiated for continued funding, professional line staff tried to neutralize the crisis atmosphere in the community for individual clients and their families. Nevertheless, the crisis took a severe toll on many Triage clients, foreshadowing the negative effects a precipitous termination would have on Triage clients and client support systems—a problem denied by Triage funders.

Termination Process

In anticipation of such an event, Triage staff had developed and submitted a proposed termination plan to the federal government 23 months before actual termination occurred. However, the federal government never acted to approve the plan, despite repeated requests from Triage staff.

Upon termination notice, Triage first addressed clients who

would require permanent institutionalization without Triage. This group required early attention to enable fiscal reimbursement criteria to be met (e.g., spend-down) and to locate appropriate nursing homes. The second client group prepared for termination were individuals capable of self-payment for their needed services. Finally, Triage terminated "multiple problem" clients who were actively dependent upon Triage case management services, did not have the financial resources to pay for services and were not eligible for entitlement programs. These clients most needed all facets of Triage program benefits and proved to be the most difficult to reenter into the traditional health care system.

Triage staff visited each client at home for a modified final reassessment and, on the basis of this reassessment, developed a continuing service plan with the client and/or client family. The service plan was then reviewed with the appropriate agencies for providing those services.

The traumatic effect of this termination process on Triage clients and their families or supporters must not be underestimated.

Post-Termination Outcomes

During its final year of operation, Triage became the manager, through contractual arrangements with the State of Connecticut, for Connecticut Community Care, Inc. (CCCI), a prototype of the Triage program without Medicare waivers. At the time that Triage ended, its seven-town region was not included among the CCCI's 83 towns. As a result of the genuine concern and personal efforts of the Speaker of the State House of Representatives and the Co-Chairman of the Legislature's Human Services Committee, legislation expanded the CCCI catchment area and provided funds to enroll a number of former high risk Triage clients into the state-sponsored program. Subsequently, some 400 ex-Triage clients met CCCI income and other eligibility criteria and now receive case management and other services. However, the hiatus that occurred while the necessary legislation was being secured resulted in a three-month loss of necessary services for many of these clients.

The case management function initiated in Triage is essentially the same in the CCCI program, but Triage's assessment/research protocol has been modified to meet CCCI operation needs and to assure uniform utilization. CCCI is actively pursuing a private market initiative and has a small number of private full-fee paying clients.

The Robert Wood Johnson Foundation funded a follow-up study to determine the impact of program termination on Triage clients. Preliminary data analysis indicates that former Triage clients, whether or not picked up by CCCI, depend heavily upon family and friends for continued life in the community. Former clients who lack access to the CCCI brokerage system are experiencing great difficulty in getting consistent, reliable care apart from physician and pharmaceutical services. For them, the same health care system delivery problems they and their families experienced prior to Triage returned in full force. Clearly, the problems facing the elderly, their families, and providers of direct health care service which prompted the original Triage experiment in 1974 continue to much the same degree. A Triage-type health resource management system, viewed post hoc, is proving to have been a worthwhile investment for both consumers and providers of long term care services.

Policy Implications

It is important to understand the historical framework of the demonstration method under which the Triage project was developed and operated. Not only was the knowledge of the needs of the long term care population very limited when Triage began, but the commitment of the majority of health care research and demonstration efforts was limited to a three-year time frame. We now know it requires at least a decade to observe significant changes in the long term care population.

Since operational start-up for demonstration projects requires at least a year, with another for winding down, the three-year time frame obviates steady state results regarding outcome validity. Were it not for the negotiation process to approve Triage's research design, the project's initial funding period would have been limited to three years.

When Triage began, its federal project officers, interested and committed to long term care, were particularly anxious that program implementation occur in a reasoned fashion. Even as Triage evolved, however, the federal view of the project altered considerably. After the Department of Health, Education and Welfare (now Health and Human Services) reorganized and the Health Care Financing Administration (HCFA) began, focused interest and knowledge in the long term care arena decreased significantly. The growing discontinuity in federal monitoring of the project, due to political administration changes as well as new public policy inconsistencies, created tremendous difficulties in implementing the Triage research and demonstration effort during both grant periods.

At the end of its second grant period, federal justification for the termination of Triage was simply that since the project had existed longer than any other, nothing new could be learned from it. This decision was made without any analysis of Triage II information—a more cogent and consistent data base on the impact of targeting a high risk population than any other at the federal level. The Health Care Financing Administration (HCFA) was disinterested in the public-private initiative Triage had designed for its proposed continuation—testing ways of involving third-party payors in the long term care reimbursement process—and viewed Triage as an experiment solely to test the effectiveness of home care over institutional care. In actuality, Triage was to test a delivery mechanism that offered a coordinated continuum of care using a single funding source without a predisposition toward either home care or institutional care.

In direct contrast to HCFA's position, the private sector showed significant interest in Triage at this time. Private third-party payors were interested in pursuing both continued client data collection and information on the impact and costs of the Triage alternative long term care service delivery system. Congress, too, began to recognize that data from Triage and other comparable long term care projects could be used to address the legislative and budgetary issues surrounding long term care. To that end, Congress inserted specific language into the Conference Report of the 1981 Omnibus Reconciliation Act urging the Secretary of Health and Human Services to review and continue those long term care research and demonstration projects which were meeting their goals and objectives (HR 3982 Conference Report, 1981, p. 968).

Ironically, the National Channeling Demonstration—a federal demonstration using a Triage case management prototype—was being initiated in ten states while Triage's termination was occurring. The federal government's failure to utilize Triage and other existing long term care demonstrations as a basis for new program implementation is evidence of a disturbing, turf-oriented long term care interest. Consultation from these operational long term care demonstrations was actively discouraged by federal officials during the National Channeling Demonstration planning phase. Rather than serving to connect previous long term care research efforts into a policy related continuum of knowledge, this demonstration appears to be establishing itself as yet another island of research inquiry.

The concept of targeting high risk individuals for long term care services has proven to be considerably more complex than many would care to admit. The effectiveness of projects such as Triage lies in their capacity to procure and coordinate a variety of medical and non-medical health services not only to control costs and utilization but to moderate the volatility of changes in individual health status. This volatility results from the uneven focus of acute, episodic care and the general inability to relate acute care services to long term maintenance care.

Triage found that compartmentalizing the older adult into high risk targeting situations is an inefficient, insensitive use of resources. Health care delivery and reimbursement systems must be restructured to view the older adult as having chronic health conditions that become exacerbated by acute episodes. The concept of the consumer must also be expanded to include the older adult and his/her support system.

While the need to explore all areas of long term health care is important, time-limited demonstration projects are inherently dangerous to the older adult with chronic health problems. The impact of a service organization closing its doors in a community leaves a vacuum that is often difficult to fill. The traditional target group—the frail elderly—depend upon specific services rendered by both providers of care and project case management staff and are adversely affected by disruption in the continuum of care. The element of risk to clients becomes apparent when services covered in a unique research effort must cease. Costs to individuals and to reimbursers may escalate when the client again becomes a victim of traditional reimbursement policies with their focus on high cost services in institutional settings.

The problems which motivated the Triage project and other long term care experiments will only be remedied incrementally. The short term political concerns which dominate transient federal administrations must be put aside and national policymakers must begin to understand that health systems that do a good job of caring are not at odds with the need for cost containment.

REFERENCES

Connecticut Statewide Health Coordinating Council. *Connecticut state health plan 1979-1983.* Hartford, CT: Author, April 23, 1979.

Health Care Financing Administration. Personal communication between Zachary Y. Dyckman and HCFA staff, 1982.

Kahn, R. L., Goldfarb, A. I., Pollack, M., and Gerber, T. E. The relationship of mental and physical status in institutionalized aged persons. *American Journal of Psychiatry,* 1960, *117,* 120-124.

Katz, S., Ford, A. B., Moskowitz, R. W., Jackson, B., and Jaffee, M. Studies of illness in the aged: The index of ADL, a standardized measure of biological and psychosocial function. *Journal of the American Medical Association,* 1963, *185,* 914-919.

Lawton, M. P., & Brody, E. M. Assessment of older people: Self-maintaining and instrumental activities of daily living. *The Gerontologist,* 1969, *9,* 179-186.

U.S. Congress, House. *HR 3982 conference report,* 1981.

Weed, L. L. *Medical records, medical evaluation, and patient care.* Cleveland: Case Western Reserve University Press, 1971.

PART III

BRINGING IT TOGETHER—
A BEGINNING

Introduction

In Part III of this monograph, the focus moves from individual projects to the groups as a whole to identify common and differentiating elements in program characteristics and research findings and to explore policy implications. Chapter 10, after briefly reviewing community-based long term care demonstrations that could not be included in Part II of this monograph, provides a framework by which the projects in Part II can be compared and arrays these projects in terms of this model. Chapter 11 focuses on what has been learned from the projects collectively by analyzing their research findings. In addition, gaps in knowledge are identified, some of the dilemmas in research on community-based projects are discussed, and an alternative to the time-limited demonstration approach is presented. Finally, Chapter 12 looks at the policy environment of these projects. It outlines the impact these projects already have had in reshaping public policy related to the delivery and reimbursement of long term care, explores the tradeoffs inherent in various policy options, and offers recommendations.

Chapter 10

Comparing the Demonstrations: A Review of Similarities and Differences

Rick T. Zawadski, PhD

The eight demonstrations described in Part II of this monograph represent a subset of some of the better known long term care demonstrations which have been operating long enough to have some data but are recent enough so that key staff in the demonstration are still available. Before focusing on these projects to compare their characteristics and outcomes, it is important to acknowledge and describe, albeit briefly, some of the other community-based long term care demonstrations that could not be included in this monograph.

OTHER LONG TERM CARE DEMONSTRATIONS

While not fitting within the boundaries of this monograph, there currently are three other major demonstration programs that are worth special mention: the Medicare Capitation Demonstration, the National Channeling Demonstration, and the Social/Health Maintenance Organization.

The Medicare Capitation Demonstration

Although their focus is on health service reimbursement rather than long term care, the Medicare Capitation demonstrations represent a shift with great importance for long term care, namely, toward prospective Medicare reimbursement. Traditionally Health Maintenance Organizations (HMOs) shied away from the aged be-

Rick T. Zawadski is Research Director, On Lok Senior Health Services, San Francisco, CA.

cause of their higher costs. When their members got older, HMOs would bill Medicare for services on a fee-for-service basis. In 1980, Medicare funded under demonstration a number of HMOs using prospective per capita payment as payment-in-full for all Medicare services. Kaiser Permanente's Medicare Plus Project in Oregon was one of these demonstrations (Greenlick; Lamb, Carpenter, Fischer, Marks, & Cooper, 1983). Kaiser found that for 95% of what Medicare would have paid for a comparable individual in that area (Average Area Per Capita Cost, or AAPCC), they could meet all Medicare obligations—including beneficiary deductibles and coinsurance—and still retain a savings.

As a follow-up on these demonstrations, legislation was included in the 1982 Tax Equity and Fiscal Responsibility Act to allow prospective per capita reimbursement. Although the AAPCC payment covers only Medicare benefits some programs, such as Kaiser, are finding it cost beneficial to provide some noncovered long term care services and are offering supplemental coverage for the expanded benefits. What started out as a health reimbursement experiment may provide a significant point of entry for Medicare reimbursement of long term care.

National Channeling Demonstration

Another interesting demonstration project is Channeling, a multi-state long term care demonstration derived from the case management service coordination pioneered by Triage. However, unlike Triage it does not include hospitals and nursing homes in the continuum of care. The National Channeling Demonstration is attempting to test whether coordinated service delivery systems, some of which control payment for service and others which rely on the traditional payment system, can serve the needy in an appropriate and cost-effective manner. The project is to be evaluated by Mathematica, Inc. and Temple University is providing technical assistance and training to the sites. While the project has not been in operation long enough for inclusion in this monograph, it is quite germane in that it represents a multi-site demonstration of coordinated community-based long term care. Unfortunately, research design issues have played a dominant and prescriptive role in the Channeling demonstrations, limiting the individual sites' flexibility and adaptability and rendering the demonstration somewhat artificial.

Social/Health Maintenance Organization

An even newer demonstration project is the Social/Health Maintenance Organization (S/HMO) demonstration arranged and coordinated through Brandeis University. The S/HMO applies the principles of the HMO to the general older population, and incorporates, at least in theory, social as well as medical services. As with Channeling, the S/HMO demonstration involves multiple sites in different states; but unlike the Channeling demonstration, Brandeis has emphasized the selection of established service providers and has given them considerable freedom and autonomy to develop programs within the broad capitation-based reimbursement guidelines of the demonstration.

The S/HMO concept has significant potential, if practical decisions made in implementation do not prove to be too problematic. For example, the sites agreed to accept the AAPCC for Medicare—that is, what Medicare now pays for primarily medical services—for an expanded package of service which supposedly includes social and supportive services. The sites are likely to find it difficult within these budget constraints to provide the social and supportive services so important to prevent deterioration and so integral to comprehensive long term care. To complicate matters, three of the four sites have well-established reputations for serving the impaired aged. This history, in conjunction with the greater propensity of the service needy to join a comprehensive service program, is likely to result in higher than average costs. To compensate, the projects have developed a queueing or quota system for different categories of enrollees and are negotiating for Medicaid reimbursement and a higher Medicare rate for the impaired. Unfortunately these changes complicate what conceptually was an administratively simple risk-based system.

COMPARISON OF DEMONSTRATIONS IN PART II

Part II's individual descriptions of the demonstration projects in some ways show the projects to be quite alike. They all, for example, have been made possible with waivers from health care programs, e.g., Medicare or Medicaid. They all expand the scope of services normally covered by these funding programs and integrate to some degree social and supportive services with medical services.

Further, all focus on a frail population. Finally, all the programs hope to reduce or contain hospital and/or nursing home utilization and, implicitly if not explicitly, to control the cost of long term care.

Nevertheless, the programs are very different from one another. They are of varying "ages" and operate from a range of organizational bases. Some directly provide services while others primarily authorize reimbursement. Some include a full range of services (acute and skilled nursing facility care, plus community out-of-home and in-home services) while others include only community-based services. Some actually make payment for services while others work primarily with cost estimates.

Further, the projects differ in the type and degree of integration they achieve in their efforts to mold long term care services into a more comprehensive, more coordinated SYSTEM of long term care. Four types of integration can be distinguished: (1) service population integration; (2) structural service integration; (3) functional service integration; and (4) fiscal integration. Each of these types is defined below.

Figure 1 has been constructed to allow a systematic, if brief, comparison of the eight demonstrations presented in Part II. In addition to each project's approach to the four areas of integration, other descriptive information is provided. That information includes data about the age of the project (i.e., operating dates) and the organizational context in which it operates (or type of sponsoring organization).

Project Age and Organizational Context

The average age of the demonstrations considered in Part II is four years. However, the operating dates for the projects, shown in Figure 1, provide a distorted picture, implying that these programs have sprung quickly to life and are neatly bounded demonstrations of approximately the same length. Triage started as long ago as 1974 while two others began as recently as 1980 (Community Long Term Care and Home Care Project). In some instances, these demonstrations represent continuations and further development of past efforts in long term care. Mount Zion had developed an innovative home care program decades before the current demonstration project and had a grant in 1975 for an adult day health center; On Lok had its first demonstration grant in 1972 and the organization's present CCODA project developed as part of a continuous evolution from that first project; Monroe County, New York, where AC-CESS developed, had been at the forefront of long term care improvement for 25 years prior to ACCESS. The fact that some of the projects are no longer operating on a demonstration basis

Figure 1
PROGRAM CHARACTERISTICS

Project	Developed	Operating Dates (under waivers)	Sponsoring Organization	Structural Service Integration
ACCESS (New York)	1976	12/77 -	Private nonprofit community organiza-tion; county and state contracts	SNF; out-of-home community care; In-home communi-ty care
ALTERNATIVE HEALTH SERVICES (Georgia)	1976	7/76 - 6/80	State Dept of Medical Assistance	Out-of-home community, In-home communi-ty care
COMMUNITY LONG TERM CARE (South Carolina)	1978	7/80 -	State Dept of Social Services (State Medicaid agency)	Out-of-home community, In-home communi-ty care
HOME CARE PROJECT (New York)	1979	12/80 -	NYC Dept of Aging Adminis-tration health & social serv-ice provider	Out-of-home community, In-home communi-ty care
NURSING HOME WITHOUT WALLS (New York)	1978	10/79 -	Private nonprofit com-munity organiza-tion; State administered	Out-of-home community, In-home communi-ty care
PROJECT OPEN (California)	1978	8/80 - 6/83	Private nonprofit hospital working with consortium	Out-of-home community, In-home communi-ty care
ON LOK CCODA (California)	1972	2/79 -	Private nonprofit adult day health program	Acute; SNF; out-of-home community, In-home communi-ty care
TRIAGE (Connecticut)	1974	2/74 - 12/81	Private nonprofit community organization	Acute; SNF; out-of-home community, In-home communi-ty care

Figure 1 (cont'd)

PROJECT	Functional Service Integration	Fiscal Integration	Population Served	Explicit Primary Objective
ACCESS (New York)	Preauthorization screening; case management	Funded by Medicaid, Medicare in 1980	18+; at risk	Reduce acute & SNF utilization; more appropriate home care & SNF utilization
ALTERNATIVE HEALTH SERVICES (Georgia)	Preauthorization screening; case management	Funded by Medicaid; authorized eligibility for benefits	50+; Medicaid SNF/ICF eligible	Prevent or delay SNF utilization
COMMUNITY LONG TERM CARE (South Carolina)	Preauthorization screening; case management	Funded by Medicaid and Medicare; authorizes service and payment up to 75% of SNF costs	18+; Impaired in areas of ADL and/or ICF/SNF level of care	Reduce or delay SNF placement
HOME CARE PROJECT (New York)	Case management	Funded by Medicare; authorizes service and payment	65+; homebound Medicare Part B	Contain costs for services to homebound; prevent or delay SNF utilization
NURSING HOME WITHOUT WALLS (New York)	Case management; some service delivery, with some sites approaching consolidation	Funded by Medicaid, private pay; authorizes service and payment to 75% of ICF/SNF costs	Any age; SNF/ICF eligible	Reduce SNF utilization; reduce fragmentation in home care services
PROJECT OPEN (California)	Case management; some service delivery	Funded by Medicare; authorized service and payment	65+; difficulty living and/or functioning independently; Medicare eligible	Reduce hospital & SNF utilization; inhibit decline in functional status; contain costs
ON LOK CCODA (California)	Consolidation; direct service delivery	Funded by Medicare, Medicaid and copayment in 1983; authorizes service and pays directly	55+; SNF/ICF certified	Contain costs; provide appropriate health services; reduce hospital & SNF utilization; improve functioning
TRIAGE (Connecticut)	Case management	Funded by Medicare, private pay in 1979; authorized service and payment	60+; at risk	Provide appropriate health care services; improve functioning

(Triage and Alternative Health Services) is discussed further in Chapter 12.

What is important to note is that these demonstrations have a developmental history either through the organization or key project staff that predates the specific demonstration. It is unlikely that any of the demonstrations could have operated a service system without that background and base.

Many of the projects are run by private nonprofit community organizations, some developed specifically for the project, although auspices range from a hospital (Project OPEN) to state government departments (Alternative Health Services and Community Long Term Care). Background and perspectives of the parent organization may influence the shape of the demonstration. For example, Mount Zion Hospital's long history of geriatric services and working relationships with community agencies can be linked to its choice of a consortium approach and brokerage model.

There are advantages and disadvantages to each arrangement. A freestanding organization focusing on the demonstration has the autonomy to act and adapt with singularity of purpose and to direct all organizational resources to the demonstration. A demonstration affiliated with an existing organization has the advantage of the resources of that organization—its history, reputation, access to a service population, administrative services, and a larger financial base.

Objectives

The projects are most similar in terms of their objectives, although there are some differences in the objectives projects list as primary; and these primary objectives have a big role in determining project direction and outcomes. In an attempt to provide more appropriate and cost-effective services as needed, most of the projects have as a primary objective the reduction or control of hospital and/or nursing home utilization. In addition, a few of the projects explicitly aim to improve or at least to maintain the functional status of those they serve (Triage, Project OPEN, and On Lok CCODA) and a few emphasize the impact on life satisfaction of participants.

Service Population Integration

Service population integration refers to the incorporation of various client groups into the program. Projects may intend to serve a very broad clientele or target their services quite narrowly, using either formal restrictions or de facto operational means. Projects may target a subset of the aged population using such criteria as age, financial entitlements or functional level of need. In one project, the aged are defined as those 50 years of age and older (Alternative Health Services); in others, 55 (On Lok CCODA) or 65 and over (Project OPEN and Home Care Project). In some cases, the project is not formally restricted to serve the aged (Community Long Term Care and ACCESS serve those who are 18 years or older, Nursing Home Without Walls has no age limit). Nevertheless, the nature of services provided results in a predominantly older service population in all of the projects.

Other population restrictions are tied to the reimbursement source. A Medicare population, for example, includes those 65 years of age or older and younger persons with long term disability who have worked under the Social Security system and therefore qualify for Medicare entitlement. However, most older people can "buy-in" and qualify for Medicare reimbursement. Medicaid, on the other hand, is a health care program for the poor and has an intricate means test to determine those who are eligible. Projects typically direct and in some cases limit their programs to the people entitled to services under the funding base for which they have waivers. Alternative Health Services is limited to Medicaid eligible individuals while both Project OPEN and Home Care Project are limited to those who participate in the Medicare program.

Level of functional impairment also plays a role in targeting the population for most of these demonstrations. While all of the projects focus on a frail population, how they define "frail" varies. Some formally restrict their programs to persons certified for institutional placement; others include those who are at-risk of such placement. Frailty of the target population is defined in a number of ways: those impaired in two areas of Activities of Daily Living (Community Long Term Care); those who have difficulty living and/or functioning independently (Project OPEN); those who are homebound (Home Care Project); those who are "at risk" of institutionalization (Triage and ACCESS); those who are SNF/ICF eligible or certified (Alternative Health Services, Nursing Home Without Walls and On Lok CCODA). In certain programs, anyone actually in a skilled nursing facility must be excluded, e.g., Nursing Home Without Walls. Even without formal service population targeting, the process of selection may identify a frail population or exclude those who are too frail to seek help. Generally, people not needing services—for example, the healthy, affluent person who is over 65—do not seek help and are therefore not included in any of these programs (although they would be included in some of the other demonstrations discussed earlier in this chapter).

Structural Service Integration

Structural service integration refers to the integration of traditionally discrete services as part of the long term care systems package. Typically, community-based long term care demonstration projects integrate social and medical services into their demonstration package and expand the scope of services. However, the number and type of included services differ from project to project.

Roughly speaking, the services included fall into four general categories: acute medical care in hospital settings; skilled nursing care (in a nursing home); community in-home services (the range of health, therapeutic and supportive services provided in the client's home); and community out-of-home services (any therapeutic health or supportive service provided outside the home or institution, including transportation, adult day care, congregate meals and the like).

Projects designed as nursing home alternatives, for example, Community Long Term Care and Alternative Health Services, provide an expanded scope of community-based services so as to reduce skilled nursing placement, but generally have not included in their waiver package institutional care, such as hospital or skilled nursing care. Similarly, many of these projects omit medical services which they presume are available under normal reimbursement mechanisms. At the other end of the spectrum, waivers for a project like Triage or On Lok CCODA includes all medical, health-related and health supportive services that are required by its long term care population, including institutional care (acute and skilled nursing).

The relative emphasis on in-home community care versus out-of-home community care also varies among the projects. For example, On Lok CCODA relies heavily on out-of-home community care and uses in-home community care only when their community-based day center services are insufficient; the Home Care Project relies primarily on services provided in the home.

Projects also differ in their level of direct involvement in service delivery. ACCESS provides no direct service and contracts for or authorizes services through existing providers. Project OPEN established a consortium of existing providers with consortium members delivering most demonstration services. On Lok expanded its own service capacity and delivers almost all demonstration services through its own staff. Alternative Health Services encouraged the development of some new community services and referred its clients to one or another of the programs.

Functional Service Integration

Increased availability of services without a method of functional service integration does not necessarily improve the service system. A key ingredient in all of the demonstrations is the method of linking services to meet the individual's needs. Each project has a somewhat different approach that blends the three basic methods of functional service integration described and discussed in Chapter 1—prior authorization screening and referral; case management and brokerage; and service consolidation and direct service delivery.

The particular approach employed by a project has implications for the extent to which a project takes direct responsibility for tracking, paying for and providing a given service. For example, On Lok CCODA, a consolidated model, tracks the use of all services by its population (regardless of how these ordinarily would be reimbursed); pays for these services directly; and provides all the services either through its employees or its subcontractors. On the other hand, Community Long Term Care, through pre-authorization screening and case management, tracks only community and home care services; does not directly provide or reimburse services; but does authorize reimbursement of services for up to 75% of the cost of service in a long term care facility. Triage, through case management, tracked all services, although none were provided directly, and authorized reimbursement, although it did not actually reimburse.

Fiscal Integration

Fiscal integration refers to the extent to which the different funding sources involved in the reimbursement of long term care have been linked or integrated in a particular demonstration. Traditionally long term care has suffered from barriers resulting from multiple funding sources with different objectives. Such barriers include service limitations (types and levels), entitlement restrictions (means tests), paperwork requirements (multiple reporting systems), and other cumbersome policies such as fee-for-service billing.

Demonstration projects implicitly and in some cases explicitly integrate funding sources in the process of integrating services, thereby removing some of the reimbursement barriers. When the scope of services normally reimbursed by a funding source is expanded, reimbursement for all the included services—the usually covered and the newly included—becomes integrated. Similarly, when waivers enable usually ineligible persons to obtain services—for example, the not-yet-poor to receive Medicaid-reimbursed services or those not qualified for Medicare to participate in Medicare-funded projects, funding for services for this population becomes more integrated.

The demonstration projects vary as to the degree and method for achieving fiscal integration. Many of the Medicaid demonstration programs include in their waiver package an expanded means test to broaden participation, e.g., Community Long Term Care extends community Medicaid services to individuals who otherwise would have been eligible for coverage only if they were in a nursing home. Other projects have waivers that allow a percentage of persons normally not included for that reimbursement to participate, e.g., up to 10% of those in On Lok's program need not be eligible for Medicare. Some projects have taken an even more direct approach by obtaining reimbursement from multiple funding sources in order to include multiple populations, e.g., ACCESS now has both Medicaid and Medicare reimbursement, as does Community Long Term Care.

While all of the demonstrations explicitly or implicitly sought to control costs, the method of reimbursement and the degree of control available over reimbursement influence the projects' incentive and ability to control costs. The amount of control over reimbursement and the exercise of this control varies for the projects. Alternative Health Services has no control over reimbursement. In most of the other projects, service and reimbursement are authorized by the project often with a cap on the amount authorized (Community Long Term Care, Nursing Home Without Walls, and ACCESS). Moving toward further control, On Lok CCODA functions essentially as a fiscal intermediary, actually paying for all services delivered.

Methods of reimbursement range from the traditional fee-for-service basis to cost reimbursement. Most projects receive or authorize reimbursement on a traditional fee-for-service basis at the going rate; others are reimbursed for their costs. A prospective per diem rate is being tried on a limited basis by ACCESS for some nursing home care under its 222 Medicare project. Prospective capitation payment for comprehensive long term care with provider assumption of risk is a new, yet untried method but it is soon to be undertaken by at least one project (On Lok CCODA).

All of these program differences impact on the projects' research findings. In the next chapter, the impacts of the areas discussed above will be explored.

REFERENCE

Greenlick, M. R., Lamb, S. J., Carpenter, T. M., Jr., Fischer, T. S., Marks, S. D., & Cooper, W. J. Kaiser-Permanente's Medicare Plus Project: A successful Medicare prospective payment demonstration. *Health Care Financing Review,* 1983, *4,* 85-97.

Chapter 11

Research in the Demonstrations: Findings and Issues

Rick T. Zawadski, PhD

In Part II of this monograph, the individual demonstration projects described their service programs and populations and presented some data on outcomes. The next step is to abstract from these individual experiences the general principles and relationships which appear consistently across projects. Where project findings are inconsistent it is useful to begin exploring possible explanations for these differences as they relate to the input variables. This chapter cuts across the different demonstration projects, compares their findings, identifies methodological problems inherent in the study of different factors, discusses some of the broader issues in the study of community-based systems of long term care, and proposes an alternative approach to community-based research and demonstration in long term care.

CROSS-SITE COMPARISON OF FINDINGS

The community-based long term care projects described in Part II represent individual experiments or demonstrations. While the findings of these projects are interesting in and of themselves, it is important to assess the generalizability of their experiences by comparing some of the data and results across projects. This comparison represents a form of replication but also provides a base for identifying important similarities, differences and, in some cases, moderators accounting for those differences.

Cross-site project descriptions and comparisons have been done in the past. In June of 1980 an issue of *The Gerontologist* was devoted to long term care, and five demonstration projects were included. Unfortunately, the projects did not use a common format, making comparison difficult. In addition, there was no attempt to integrate the information across the different demonstrations. Later in that year, the Urban Institute released a working paper representing a comparative analysis of long term care demonstrations and evaluations (Stasson & Holahan, 1981). Their analysis reviewed demonstrations of community-wide coordinated care programs, adult day health care programs, and in-home services. In December of 1982, the Government Accounting Office (GAO) also released a report describing and comparing some of the research and demonstration projects in community-based long term care. Both the Urban Institute and the GAO cross-site analyses focused heavily on design and methodological issues and sought to derive clear conclusions on complicated areas such as impacts on institutionalization, costs and effectiveness. Unfortunately, neither of these efforts took the next step to look more closely at the demonstrations to identify some of the program characteristics which may have accounted for differences in findings; nor did these analyses consider the practical issues in program start-up and their impacts on costs and outcomes.

Berkeley Planning Associates is now under contract with the Health Care Financing Administration to study fifteen HCFA-funded long term care demonstration projects. Unlike the other cross-site evaluations, this project is gathering some client information across a number of the projects and is attempting to identify and, to some extent, quantify some of the common and differentiating elements in the demonstrations. Unfortunately, because providers are not playing as big a role in defining these factors as originally proposed, some of the practical issues in program implementation are somewhat underrepresented. Working papers from the BPA study have been prepared, and the final report is due in 1984.

COMPARISON OF DATA FROM PROJECTS IN PART II

Like the other cross-site efforts, this section seeks to compare projects. However, the present analysis focuses on the similarities and differences across programs and looks to the qualitative differences in the demonstrations themselves to explain the consistencies and inconsistencies in findings. While this analysis does not take the desirable but currently impossible step of coordinating and integrating client information from all the projects into a single database, it does use a program-based policy orientation in the interpretation of project findings. With its policy orientation, the focus is on broad policy issues such as cost control, institutional substitution, and impacts on functional status. With its program-based emphasis, however, these issues are examined through the eyes of the program developers and providers. Thus, the practical issues and constraints are identified and incorporated in the interpretation of the cross-site data.

The demonstrations described in Part II are not, nor do they contend to be, the definitive studies of certain service models. They are pioneering research projects, representing new models of service delivery, with data reflecting early outcomes and changes in the state-of-the-art. The eight demonstration projects used different research designs, different data collection systems and focused on different variables in assessing the impacts of their programs. To complicate matters further, some of these projects are in different phases of analysis; therefore, all data are not yet available on certain issues or measures—especially those relating to changes over time in service patterns, cost or functional status.

Since the individual projects were asked to give just a brief summary of their research findings in their articles for Part II, they could not go into great detail about their methods, design, variables and analyses. Rather than evaluate in detail the methodological issues and alternative explanations relevant to each project, the following summary presents the findings and conclusions of the various chapters side by side, highlighting some of the similarities and differences. Three outcome areas are looked at: cost, service, and effectiveness. In Figure 1, the research designs used by each of the projects are summarized along with their service and cost findings. Since there was little commonality among the projects in their choice of effectiveness measures, these findings were not included in the figure but are discussed below. There are methodological and analytical questions that could be and indeed should be raised, and some of these broader issues will be discussed in the last part of this chapter.

Cost

Cost—whether it be health care cost, public sector cost, or total cost—represents the key policy issue today. While public hearings may address issues of quality of care, such an intangible issue recedes in the back room discussions regarding the cost impacts of various service alternatives. Cost represents an easily understood bottom line for comparing various alternatives. Unfortunately,

Figure 1

RESEARCH FINDINGS BY PROJECT

Project	Research Design	Acute Care Services	Skilled Care Services	Community Services
ACCESS (New York)	Quasi-experimental non-equivalent groups	Lower ACF back-up days	Shift in SNF population	Higher utilization of home health services
ALTERNATIVE HEALTH SERVICES (Georgia)	Experimental random assignment	Not reported	No difference in SNF admissions	Not reported
COMMUNITY LONG TERM CARE (South Carolina)	Experimental random assignment	Not reported	Lower SNF admissions	Not reported
HOME CARE PROJECT (New York)	Quasi-experimental matched group comparison	Length of stay in ACF decreased	No difference in SNF admissions	Not reported
NURSING HOME WITHOUT WALLS (New York)	Quasi-experimental comparable groups	Not reported	Not reported	Not reported
PROJECT OPEN (California)	Experimental random assignment	Lower ACF admissions	Lower SNF utilization	More comprehensive range of services; pattern of more community services
ON LOK CCODA (California)	Quasi-experimental matched individual comparison	Lower ACF utilization	Lower SNF utilization	Higher utilization of community services
TRIAGE (Connecticut)	Quasi-experimental matched group comparison	Higher ACF utilization	Lower SNF utilization	Higher utilization of home health services

Figure 1 (cont'd)

Project	Informal Supports	Cost Savings	Cost Redistribution
ACCESS (New York)	Informal supports maintained	Medicaid costs increased at a lower rate	Medicaid costs lower for SNF, higher for home care
ALTERNATIVE HEALTH SERVICES (Georgia)	Not reported	Higher costs, but lower than comparable SNF stay	Not specified
COMMUNITY LONG TERM CARE (South Carolina)	Not reported	Not reported	Not reported
HOME CARE PROJECT (New York)	Informal supports maintained	Not reported	Not reported
NURSING HOME WITHOUT WALLS (New York)	Informal supports appear to have increased	Average expenditures approximately one-half comparable cost of SNF	Not specified
PROJECT OPEN (California)	Decline of social network inhibited	Average monthly savings of $139 per participant	Not specified
ON LOK CCODA (California)	Informal supports maintained	Average monthly savings of $193 per participant	From inpatient to community care
TRIAGE (Connecticut)	Not reported	No overall savings	From SNF to other categories

while it is easy to ask what the cost is, it is far more difficult to compare costs across projects validly because of geographic variation, inflationary changes over time, and differences in costing methods and cost items included. Although total costs cannot be compared, cost findings can.

Six of the eight demonstrations report information on cost. At first glance the findings appear somewhat inconsistent, with three projects showing cost savings, two showing no impacts, and one showing a cost increase.

New York's Nursing Home Without Walls Project reported cost

data showing alternative health service costs to be half the charge for a nursing home day. This kind of savings was to be expected because of that project's cap—the cost for alternative community services for individuals participating in the demonstration could not exceed 75% of the cost of institutional care. It is difficult to assess total cost impacts of this demonstration, however, because other costs—hospitalization, physician services, etc.—are not included. In addition, high-cost individuals, those whose service cost in community settings would exceed the 75% limitation, are excluded, presumably referred to nursing homes. Since all of Nursing Home Without Walls' participants are required to meet eligibility requirements for nursing home placement, the data from this project do suggest that some portion of those qualifying for institutional care can be served in the community at a cost below nursing home rates.

Two other projects reported cost savings. Mount Zion's Project OPEN reported an average savings of $139 per participant per month for health care costs, savings due in large part to reductions in hospital costs. On Lok's CCODA looked at total public sector cost, including health expenditures and other costs such as Supplemental Security Income (SSI) and housing subsidies, and found total cost to be 12% lower for the intervention group (average savings of $193 per participant per month). For On Lok the lower hospitalization and skilled nursing facility utilization more than offset the higher costs for additional community-based services.

For two projects, Triage and Monroe County's ACCESS, there was no reduction in total cost. What these projects did report was some reduction in skilled nursing costs. For ACCESS this was offset by increased community costs, primarily for in-home service expenditures; for Triage, cost was redistributed to community services and hospital care. As with the other demonstrations, it is unclear whether there would be long-term cost benefits provided through the prophylactic benefits of community services.

Georgia's Alternative Health Services was the only demonstration project to report overall higher health care costs. The authors of that report note that for the very frail, e.g., those likely to go into skilled nursing facilities, the cost of the expanded services in the community setting might be offset by savings in inpatient care. A possible explanation for the higher overall cost is that the population may have been underserved without the intervention—a possibility underscored by the fact that the project did show some reduction in mortality. In the experimental group, service needs that had previously been unmet may have been identified, and an appropriate level of services provided. As a result, savings in inpatient care for those diverted into community services were offset by increases in inpatient care in acute and skilled facilities for those legitimately requiring such services. A more appropriate level of service utilization would result, in the short run, in lower mortality and higher costs for some individuals; while some of the longer terms savings in higher cost services due to preventive measures would require more time to manifest themselves.

Thus, taken together, these apparently inconsistent results are not all that inconsistent. All of the projects being demonstrations of community service programs do have increased costs related to additional services. In some cases, these additional services replaced other more costly medical services, e.g., hospitalization or skilled nursing care. In other cases, however, the services seemed to represent additional expense. This additional expense may have resulted in a higher quality of care—perhaps accounting for Georgia's lower mortality rate—or may have future benefits in preventing deterioration and higher cost.

Another point that comes through clearly is that the greatest cost savings are achieved when projects focus on individuals who are likely to be "high cost," that is, when projects target a very frail population. A number of the demonstrations noted the importance of targeting (e.g., see Chapter 3). The more frail the population, the higher the expected expenditures, and the greater the opportunity for cost savings. Thus, projects like On Lok and Nursing Home Without Walls have the greatest likelihood of cost savings, while programs such as Triage, which aim at an at-risk population with lower expected cost, have less opportunity for savings (at least in the short run). These latter projects, given a longer time frame, might show cost benefits of more comprehensive coordinated preventive care. Unfortunately, research designs and models used today do not afford the opportunity to assess such longer term benefits of more innovative long term care.

An interesting point emerged which relates to the "woodwork phenomenon." This phenomenon refers to the belief that there exists a large group of people living in the community who need and are entitled to additional services, but who are going without them because these services are unavailable or because available services (e.g., nursing homes) are unappealing; increasing availability of community-based services may draw these underserved people out of the "woodwork," thereby increasing costs. However, Triage's frailest participants who remained in the community used less nursing home days but incurred much higher hospital and in-home service costs. The same was true for On Lok's Comparison group.

Another "closet fear" about cost is related to longevity. If new service programs prolong life, costs may increase. With new developments in medical technology, life can be maintained for longer and longer periods; but at what cost and for whose benefit? Following that line of thought through to its logical conclusion may result in arguments for euthanasia. This basic "cost benefit" issue is a growing moral dilemma that must soon be addressed by society. In the acute care medical setting the emphasis has traditionally been on maintaining life at almost any cost. On the other hand, long term care providers, especially community-based providers, have been particularly close to this dilemma and are increasingly focusing on the maximization of quality of life, not quantity of life. One example is their support of the living will, which reflects not just a sense of societal cost responsibility but a strong appreciation for the dignity of the individual.

One caveat that must be raised regarding cost is the importance of analyzing *total* cost. In the past, demonstration programs have been funded usually by one source, Medicare or Medicaid, and the research designs have emphasized costs borne by these programs, e.g., Medicare projects focused on controlling hospital costs and Medicaid projects focused on controlling nursing home costs. Service need, however, is fluid: some hospitalization, some skilled nursing and some community services may always be needed, and the capacity of one service to take the overflow of another should not be underestimated. For example, nursing home availability can reduce hospitalization; availability of community services can result in lower nursing home or acute hospitalization. If our cost criteria focus only on one part of this fluid system, it is quite easy to miss impacts in related areas. Future cost analyses of alternative health systems must look at all public sector costs: the many and varied medical costs as well as the social, supportive, and even the added costs of community versus nursing home living such as housing and cash subsidies.

Impacts on Service Utilization

Most of the projects had as a primary objective the reduction of institutional days, either skilled nursing, acute hospital or both. It was hypothesized by these projects that savings in these high-cost service units would offset the increase in community-based service units. The hospital day represents the "mega-buck" in health care today, typically the highest cost element in a service package, with 70% of all Medicare expenditures going to hospital care.

Hospital utilization. Hospital use reflects both the number of hospitalizations and length of stay: It may be affected by special factors such as back-up days in the hospital during which the patient is awaiting SNF placement. The different demonstrations have influenced one or more of these factors. Mount Zion's Project OPEN reported a lower number of acute hospital admissions. New York City's Home Care Project reported decreases in length of stay in acute facilities. Monroe County's ACCESS found lower hospital back-up days. On Lok's CCODA in its Comparative Study found a reduction in overall hospital utilization and, what is perhaps more interesting, in its Within Group Study found hospitalization for the demonstration group to be reduced by half over time. Although Georgia's Alternative Health Services examined hospital utilization, no significant differences were found. Only Triage reported higher hospitalization.

It is unfortunate that several demonstration projects did not gather information on hospital utilization. It is not surprising that most of these were demonstrations funded by Medicaid, for hospitalization is only a small part of Medicaid's cost responsibility and many of these Medicaid demonstrations focused on reduction in skilled nursing care. However, as noted above, acute hospitalization and skilled nursing care are related. A skilled nursing day can provide a cost competitive alternative to hospitalization, and reduced nursing home utilization can result in increased, more costly use of acute hospitals. It is important, therefore, that long term care demonstrations routinely gather information on hospitalization to assess direct and indirect impacts in this area.

Skilled nursing utilization. As community-based service alternatives, most of the demonstration projects sought to reduce days in the skilled nursing facility. Thus, it is not surprising that seven of the eight projects reported data on skilled nursing facility use. The eighth project, New York's Nursing Home Without Walls Program, did not have information on this item yet available. Of the seven sites reporting data, five reported some form of reduction in skilled nursing days, with only Georgia's Alternative Health Services and New York City's Home Care Project reporting no differences. ACCESS reports a shift in population admitted to skilled nursing homes. It is important to reemphasize the differences across projects in terms of population frailty. Projects like Triage and Project OPEN involve an at-risk population, while programs like Nursing Home Without Walls and On Lok serve a population qualified and/or certified for institutional placement. As a result of differences in population, the baseline rate of expected institutional use would also vary: from five to ten percent of the population in the "at-risk" demonstrations (e.g. Project OPEN)to over forty percent in the "nursing home eligible" projects (e.g. On Lok CCODA, Yordi & Waldman, 1983).

The projects seem to demonstrate that nursing home use can, at least to some extent, be controlled through use of alternative community services. The other side of this is that the better screening, assessment and care planning provided by the demonstrations may result in additional *appropriate* nursing home placements.

Community-based services. As one might expect, the reduction in hospitalization and skilled nursing days was offset by increases in community-based services. Most of the demonstrations, in effect, had the objective of substituting community-based services for inpatient services. Somewhat surprisingly, however, only four of the eight projects describe their demonstrations as impacting on utilization of community services. Triage and ACCESS report higher utilization of home health services. On Lok's CCODA reports higher utilization of community out-of-home services and a broader range of services. Mount Zion's Project OPEN shows an increase in the range of services. Despite the lack of reported data, many of the other projects, implicitly by their design, have had an impact on community services; Georgia, in its demonstration, offers day center and in-home services, and both New York's Nursing Home Without Walls Program and New York's Home Care Program offer extensive in-home services.

Informal support. Although not a formal service, questions are increasingly raised about the importance of the informal support system. There is a growing concern in this country about the role of increased public services supplanting the "free" services provided by family and friends. The data thus far suggest there is no great cause for concern. Five of the eight demonstrations were able to gather some information relating to the involvement of the informal network, and none of the five found significant differences in degree of involvement. Within projects some families were encouraged to get more involved; others became somewhat less involved; and in total there was no general effect. However, none of the projects had "increasing family involvement" as a major objective; had they focused on this area they may have been able to increase the degree of involvement.

Effectiveness: Impacts on Functional Status and Quality of Life

Cost analysis is a bottom line comparison. Cost benefit analysis looks at the services provided for each unit of funds to assess best value. A third comparison, however, is cost effectiveness or outcomes of some desired goal achieved for each cost unit.

What are the desired outcomes of these demonstrations? One can look at quantity of life, that is, mortality data, or at quality of life. A number of the demonstrations have as an explicit objective the "improvement of the quality of care or quality of life" which may mean expressions of satisfaction, improvement in health status, and improvement in functional independence. All these issues need to be addressed, and the results vary.

Of the eight projects, seven have reported data on mortality. Of these, Triage and Georgia's Alternative Health Services reported a significant reduction in mortality, although in the latter case, over a longer time period the mortality differences were not significant. Inadequate quality of care prior to the intervention could result in lower post-intervention mortality data. Since mortality was not generally affected, one might assume that existing services in this country are at least adequate to maintain life. But this assumption should be considered cautiously. The demonstration projects, even those using randomized designs, did identify and assess people in the control groups; that process of assessment identified service needs and thereby increased the likelihood that those needs were dealt with properly, an expected and appropriate artifact of a community research design.

Quality of life in its truest sense is an individual assessment. Whether a person is better off or not is based upon the individual's values, beliefs and expectations, as well as a personal assessment of the situation in light of these values. Assessment is a very complicated issue fraught with many methodological problems that are compounded by cognitive or communication impairments often present in an older population. Only three of the projects, Georgia's Alternative Health Services, Nursing Home Without Walls, and

Project OPEN, attempted to assess participants' perception of quality of life and none of these reported significant differences.

Since the individual's assessment of satisfaction is difficult to measure, a second approach would be to look at generally accepted standards of quality and to assess an individual's change on these measures. It is generally assumed that higher health and functional status is a desirable outcome, and five of the eight demonstrations reported some information in this area. Triage found improvement in some areas of functional status over time, and Project OPEN reported inhibited decline in functional status. South Carolina's Community Long Term Care and Georgia's Alternative Health Services reported no significant difference in functional status over time. On Lok reported relative improvement in many areas of functional status. Considering the projects' populations, the lack of consistent improvement in functional status is not really surprising. Many of the people being served by these demonstrations are old, impaired, and likely to deteriorate further. They are prime candidates for subsequent and additional medical problems and disabilities. For each person in the group who gets better, there is probably at least one who gets worse. Since many of the problems that are encountered in old age are irreversible, basic skills and medical status have only a little room for improvement. Thus, from a methodological perspective, functional status should be viewed not so much in terms of improvement as in terms of maintenance and retardation of further deterioration. Population data or estimates are critical, as is a longer time frame to assess these relative impacts.

ISSUES IN COMMUNITY-BASED RESEARCH

A comparison of community-based long term care research and demonstration projects brings up several broader issues which need to be addressed: research design, issues related to the intervention itself, and the role of research in demonstration projects.

Research Design

The true experimental design with pre/post data collection, double blind conditions, randomized assignment and random selection may be ideal when an intervention or treatment is well-defined, easily measured and controlled. However, in the study of community-based service programs, concerns about true experimental design seem somewhat frivolous since these service programs themselves are continuously changing and developing.

From a traditional research perspective, each of these research and demonstration projects has some methodological limitations. None of the projects, for example, randomly selected participants from a general population, a limitation on external validity (Campbell & Stanley, 1968). Randomization of participants in experimental and control groups was done in three of the projects, Georgia's Alternative Health Services, South Carolina's Community Long Term Care Program, and Mount Zion's Project OPEN. In the other demonstration communities where random assignment was not made, most projects did gather data on a comparable sample in order to assess relative impact. On Lok individually matched people entering its CCODA program with comparison group individuals from a neighboring non-covered community. New York City's Home Care Project and Nursing Home Without Walls program also used a neighboring community not involved in the demonstration to select participants and required those in the comparison group to meet the projects' admission criteria. ACCESS used comparable counties for comparison.

Randomized design in a real world setting raises a number of ethical questions (Bower & deGasparis, 1978) involving the rights of human subjects. For example, is it fair to take risks with the lives and well-being of individuals in the name of experimentation? This is particularly the case in community-based service programs where the individuals assigned to the control group are members of a "vulnerable" population, the frail at-risk elderly. Denial of services becomes problematic when the individuals are routinely assessed and service needs identified during the course of the experiment. Furthermore, where services for the elderly are deficient, community support is crucial; in such cases, randomized assignment is neither ethical or politically feasible. The expectation and, in fact, the human tendency is to respond to identified needs—whether they occur in the experimental or the control group (Yordi, Chu, Ross, & Wong, 1982).

Quite apart from the ethical and political questions, ignoring the legitimate pleas for help may have a negative impact on the individuals assigned to the control group, their willingness to participate, their compliance with the study design, and the quality of the data. These and other numerous implementation issues can overtly and subtly undermine the "purity" of the experimental design.

The Intervention

Beyond the issue of establishing an experimentally adequate control condition, there are a number of more basic problems related to the intervention itself. First, new service interventions are typically not operationally defined and the implementation of a service program often turns out to be far different from its original conceptual presentation. Second, these community service programs usually— and desirably—change over time. Information from a project's early experience leads to changes and refinements in the program. After three years, the length of a typical demonstration, a program is often just becoming efficient and effective; what was true in the first part of the demonstration is often very different in the second part. Third, the political environment in which these programs and their outside service systems operate changes over time, also affecting the control group in the traditional service setting. Finally, in instances where projects operate multiple sites, the interventions themselves generally differ across those sites raising the possibility of confounded findings and loss of crucial information. For example, in the case of the 222 studies of day care (Weissert, Wan, & Livieratos, 1979), one day care center had a heavy medical emphasis costing over $100 a day, while another was social in orientation costing under $20 a day. Rather than taking into consideration these qualitative differences in programs, the research design simply averaged them out. The research design for that study was randomized, yet seriously flawed by the homogenization of the service interventions being studied.

Role of Research

To some extent calling the projects described in Part II "research and demonstration" projects is a misnomer. For the most part, they are demonstration projects onto which a research component has been grafted more or less successfully. The emphasis on research varies across the projects as does the nature and the purpose of the research endeavor.

As suggested above, a traditional research design does not provide for the shifting sands that characterize a developing project;

rather it assumes that there will be stability and that the measures can remain constant over time. A corollary of this assumption (besides a research focus on factors that may turn out to be relatively unimportant once the program is operational) is that the research will not serve program development—findings will not be fed back to service providers. Thus, where demonstrations have been committed to a traditional research design, research may be the tail that wags the dog, inhibiting program change in order to keep the design pure.

The other extreme in the research/demonstration mix occurs when service programs make no attempt to structure their information collection efforts or to collect information systematically. The pressures for program survival are such that knowledge building tasks can easily be postponed or neglected in the crush of census-building, fund-raising and program management. The gaps in information noted in our discussion of cross-project findings may be reflections of a lower priority sometimes accorded to research.

If research is the responsibility of an outside entity, e.g., a contractor, it may be more likely to get done. However, such research may not be as likely to serve the program, that is, to focus on specific program development issues and generate information that may be used to refine program operations. A second argument that is given for outside research is independence. However, since the "outside" researchers are usually under contract to the demonstration project or are dependent on the cooperation of those projects, their independence may be an illusion.

Rather than overemphasize true experimental design, therefore, we should focus on a range of methodological limitations. We must look for better research models and methods which can build a body of knowledge for continuing program and policy development.

AN ALTERNATIVE MODEL FOR COMMUNITY-BASED RESEARCH: THE COMMUNITY LABORATORY

As a research tool, the traditional research demonstration methodology—focusing on one defined intervention—provides a relatively limited body of knowledge. It assesses primarily the overall impacts of a specific intervention while ignoring the multitude of additional questions such as what parts of the intervention have differential impacts on particular kinds of people. Yet, it is the answers to these more complicated questions that provide a base for theory and model building in the complicated sphere of human service delivery. Second, the research design for most of these demonstrations requires a static intervention and, therefore, in its strictest sense, prohibits the change in the service program, discouraging, if not preventing, any feedback of outcomes for further program development. Finally, the lack of continuity between the diverse demonstrations has actually thwarted policy change, serving to stall decision making by developing competing models and pitting them against one another for limited resources. In sum, today's time-limited research and demonstration policies do not meet the three basic objectives of research and demonstration projects: (1) to build a body of knowledge regarding the relationship between services and outcomes; (2) to develop more effective and efficient service programs; and (3) to evolve more cost-effective long term care policy.

As an alternative to time-limited research and development, existing health service expenditures can be used to support a network of "community laboratories" which would allow, and with financial incentive encourage, the evolution or organic development of more cost-effective systems of long term care. This alternative approach to service delivery development and research should incoporate the following aspects: (1) ongoing support for effective programs; (2) service delivery merged with research and training; (3) an information driven, self-adjusting service system; and (4) national networks.

Ongoing Support for Effective Programs

In the community laboratory model, as long as projects stay within present expenditure levels while meeting their populations' needs, they would receive continued financial support. Funding agencies would be responsible for determining an equitable level of reimbursement for the population chosen, whether a very frail or general population, and existing quality assurance systems would be used to ensure that quality of care is at least maintained, if not improved. These explicit incentives would encourage projects to develop more efficient means of meeting participant or individual needs.

Service Delivery Merged with Research and Training

Research and, in some cases, training would work hand in hand with service delivery to improve the quality of services and encourage the propagation of effective procedures and systems. The integration of services, research and training has been broached in other initiatives, for example, teaching nursing homes and long term care policy centers. In these other initiatives, however, the role of services takes a backseat to training and/or research functions. In the alternative model we are proposing, the service program itself would be the central driving force with research and training playing interactive and supportive roles.

Information Driven, Self-Adjusting Service System

In the proposed community laboratories, data would be routinely gathered on everyone participating in the program on an ongoing basis, and this longitudinal data set would provide the basis for service planning and decision making. With the low cost of microcomputer technology, it is possible for service providers to have information on participants' health and service history, to identify probable impacts of different interventions, and to assess on an ongoing basis the change in cost for each individual (see Zawadski & Gee, 1982). Service staff could more soundly plan services, and program management staff more readily evaluate services for future program development using within group data analysis as the preferred statistical model.

In the community laboratory model, population data and data from nonparticipants would be gathered and used to assess relative impacts, but the emphasis would be on identifying problems and assessing various solutions. Instead of using inferential analytic techniques to assess whether or not an intervention is good or bad, regression models can be used to identify the components of an intervention that result in the most change and the population for whom a particular kind of service program provides the most cost-effective alternative. Unlike the traditional research and demonstration model where service environments are almost forced to remain constant throughout the demonstration period, in the community laboratory approach change in program is seen as not only desirable but necessary. Service programs and providers would be encouraged to put forth, develop and test new service solutions as needs and techniques change over time. The research component would monitor information on different interventions to identify the effects on various population subgroups.

National Networks

Community laboratories can exist in multiple locations across the country, linked together into a network to work cooperatively towards policy change. Since community laboratories would require no new funds but only control over existing funds, there should be no limit to the number of community laboratories that develop and evolve. Since designated community laboratories would not be in competition with one another for limited dollars, they could work cooperatively—sharing findings, replicating findings in other settings, using common data sets to establish larger data bases. The more successful community laboratories could serve as training sites and technical assistance providers to spur the development of community laboratories in other areas.

* * * * *

The community laboratory model represents an information driven, rational model of long term care systems development which meets the objectives of human service research. The cross-site longitudinal data set provides an ideal tool for the researcher seeking to understand human services and the relationship between client characteristics, service delivery, and outcomes. For the service provider, techniques developed by these laboratories together with information about their outcomes would be important tools for improving service delivery and training people in effective service techniques. The development of these community laboratories in different parts of the country would represent an organic method for long term care policy change and provide a cost controlled method for propagating innovation in service delivery and more effective systems of long term health care.

REFERENCES

Alternatives to nursing home care for the frail elderly: An international symposium. *The Gerontologist,* 1980, *20.*

Bower, R., & deGasparis, P. *Ethics in social research: Protecting the interests of human subjects.* New York: Praeger Publications, 1978.

Campbell, D. J., & Stanley, J. C. *Experimental and quasi-experimental design for research.* Chicago: Rand McNally College Publishing Co., 1968.

Stassen, M., & Holahan, J. *Long-term care demonstration projects: A review of recent evaluations.* Washington, DC: Urban Institute, 1981.

U.S. General Accounting Office. *The elderly should benefit from expanded home health care but increasing these services will not insure cost reductions.* Washington, DC: Author, December 7, 1982.

Weissert, W. G., Wan, T. T. H., & Livieratos, B. B. *Effects and cost of day care and home-maker service for the chronically ill: A randomized experiment* (PHS) 79-3250). Hyatts-ville, MD: National Center for Health Services Research, August 1979.

Yordi, C. L., Chu, A. S., Ross, K. M., & Wong, S. J. Research and the frail elderly: Ethical and methodological issues in controlled social experiments. *The Gerontologist,* 1982, *22,* 72-77.

Yordi, C. L., & Waldman, J. *A comparative study of the traditional long term care system and a consolidated model of long term care: Service utilization and cost impacts.* Manuscript submitted for publication, 1983.

Zawadski, R. T., & Gee, S. *Computerized information management in long-term care: A case study* (Technical Report No. 303). San Francisco: On Lok Senior Health Services, July 1982.

Chapter 12

Policy Implications
of the Community-Based
Long Term Care Demonstrations

Rick T. Zawadski, PhD

The service programs described in Part II were funded as demonstrations to assess whether alternative approaches can improve upon the existing long term care system. An objective of the demonstration concept is for successful demonstrations to be translated into changes in reimbursement policy and practice. In this chapter, we look at the effectiveness of the demonstrations in surviving and, more than that, generating policy change, e.g., legislative mandates for long term care. Against a backdrop of the current movements in community-based long term care, an attempt is made to provide some resolution and focus for future developments.

POLICY OUTCOMES OF THE DEMONSTRATIONS

One measure of a successful demonstration is its ability to survive. Continued existence is necessary, of course, if a project is to translate its innovations into policy to be shared and adopted by others. All of the service programs described in this monograph are still in existence today, albeit in several cases in a somewhat different or revised form.

Project OPEN and New York City's Home Care Program are just ending their demonstrations; and while these programs may not continue in their present form, the organizations sponsoring these programs and the people involved in their development will continue their efforts in the field. Mount Zion Hospital has a long history of geriatric services, and even as Project OPEN is coming to an end, the hospital continues to participate in another demonstration, California's MSSP (Multipurpose Senior Service Project), and is making preparations for a new demonstration in capitated reimbursement. New York City's Department of Aging also will continue to serve the older population long after its Home Care Program demonstration ends.

When Georgia's Alternative Health Service demonstration came to an end, state legislation was enacted to extend some parts of that program statewide. This legislation was passed despite the fact that cost data from the demonstration was not favorable, contradicting the conventional wisdom that community service demonstrations will not be translated into policy and legislation unless strong experimental designs are used to prove the benefits of the intervention.

Monroe County's Project ACCESS and On Lok's CCODA have initiated new demonstrations, building upon some of their past efforts. Monroe County's long term care staff have begun a Medicare demonstration to reduce administrative stays in hospitals. On Lok is building upon the consolidated model of services it developed through the CCODA with Medicare reimbursement and is expanding its reimbursement demonstration to include assumption of risk and multiple payors—Medicare, Medicaid and private pay—reflecting a more realistic policy alternative for long term care.

The Triage project went through two phases of demonstration. While Triage as such is no longer in operation, the key developer of that program is working with the state in a similar statewide long term care endeavor. Ironically, although Triage itself was phased out, the Health Care Financing Administration and Administration on Aging have joined forces to fund the National Channeling demonstration which incorporates several facets of the Triage model.

The two remaining programs described in Part II are continuing: South Carolina is still in the midst of its demonstration, and New York's Nursing Home Without Walls program is a permanent state initiative.

These eight programs are surviving not because of the system but in spite of it. While federal health funding programs should do more than fund and administer demonstrations, they simply do not have mechanisms in place with which they can readily translate successful components of demonstration projects into ongoing policy and practice. Unfortunately, quite to the contrary, federal funding agencies view their demonstration authority as one-time and time-limited. Under these circumstances, only those programs whose political skills enable them to defy or beat the system are able to continue.

MOVEMENTS, PROGRAMS AND LEGISLATION IN COMMUNITY—BASED LONG TERM CARE

To understand community-based long term care, one must look at the movements within it to see both where it has been and where it is going. Movements are trends or directions which guide the development of a field. Typically, problems—such as inequities or inefficiency—occur in any service environment. Someone identifies the problem; solutions or alternatives are proposed; demonstrations are initiated and, in some cases, a policy change or legislation which incorporates the innovation is adopted. This legislation is usually a response by policy makers to consumers' and providers' demands for more effective systems—demands that reflect the dual concerns for quality of care and service and for cost containment. Figure 1 provides a thumbnail sketch of the major recent and proposed federal legislation affecting community-based long term care.

Moving Away From the Time-Limited Demonstration

The concept of "time-limited" is implicit in human service research and demonstration. With few research and demonstration awards available to distribute to many people, federal agencies establish a practice of trying to give no one more than one. Typically, programs are funded for three years; and projects are expected to institute their programs, operate them at optimal levels immediately, analyze the findings, and close the program down. The agencies overseeing research and demonstration projects argue that if a demonstration is successful it should be translated into policy; therefore, second or extended demonstrations are unnecessary and inappropriate.

This perspective is rather naive. Even when legislation follows the demonstration programs, it takes more than three years to establish that legislation. More typically, at the end of three years the service program has just become fully operational and is only then approaching an effective operational stage. The present system of time-limited demonstrations, in effect, serves as a stalling mechanism. It diverts the energy of motivated people who are really concerned about finding more effective solutions to the long term care problem. This technique, intentionally or not, serves to impede real policy change.

Time-limited funding of community-based long term care demon-

Figure 1

RECENT AND PROPOSED FEDERAL LEGISLATION
ON COMMUNITY-BASED LONG TERM CARE

RECENT LEGISLATION

Omnibus Reconciliation Act of 1980

- Authorizes Medicare reimbursement for comprehensive outpatient rehabilitation facilities (CORFs) to provide comprehensive long term care services.

Omnibus Reconciliation Act of 1981

- Section 2175 increases flexibility in state Medicaid programs to control
  costs through competitive bidding and 1915 waivers for case management
  systems of long term care.
- Section 2176 authorizes states to substitute home and community-based
  services for institutional long term care when appropriate and cost-
  effective (also known as The Community Care Act).

The Tax Equity and Fiscal Responsibility Act of 1982

- Section 114 authorizes eligible organizations to enter into either cost-
  based reimbursement or risk-sharing contracts with Medicare for the
  provision of long term care services.
- Section 123 allows Medicare beneficiaries to receive extended care services
  without meeting a three-day prior hospitalization requirement.

PROPOSED LEGISLATION

Use of Block Grants (Example: S1539, 98th Congress Home and Community-Based
Service for the Elderly and Disabled Act)

- Encourages states to develop medical, social and supportive services to
  prevent unnecessary institutionalization.
- Directs states to assess the need for community-based services, develop
  methods of client assessment and, in response, recommend cost-effective
  services.
- Amends the Public Health Service Act.

Integration of Medicaid with Other Programs (Except Medicare) (Example:
S1540, 98th Congress Community Health Care Service Act of 1983)

- Aspires to coordinate programs currently funded by the Public Health Act,
  the Older Americans Act and state Medicaid programs.
- Allows states to implement either brokerage or consolidated programs
  emphasizing participant assessment and reassessment.
- Amends Title XIX of the Social Security Act allowing states to implement
  home health care programs for Medicaid recipients.

Part D Medicare (Example: S1244, 98th Congress Senior Citizens Independent
Community Care Act)

- Provides for the long term care needs of the elderly only via a new
  Medicare "Part D."
- Allows states to administer program following a four-year trial period by
  four states.
- Is similar to S1539 in legislative intent but funded through Medicare, not
  federal grants.

Title XXI of the Social Security Act

- Combines services currently provided for by Medicare, Medicaid and Title XX
  to eliminate some fragmentation and duplication.

strations nullifies two critical ingredients for the development of better long term care systems: leadership and skill building. One can only wonder how far the space effort would have gone had it been funded as a series of separate discrete demonstrations, with the team disbanded every three years to be replaced by another which had to be trained before it could move forward.

An interesting alternative to the time-limited demonstration has been put forth in the 1981 Omnibus Reconciliation Act. That act established a new Medicaid demonstration waiver authority—1915 A, B, and C—that not only encourages the development of community-based services, but also allows for demonstrations without formal time limitations and research requirements. By allowing two-year funding with unlimited renewals, the ''1915'' community service demonstration waivers provide an alternative to the ''1115'' time-limited research and demonstration waiver. The 1115 waivers have funded most of the innovations in long term care but have been restrictive because of their time limitation, usually one year with up to two extensions for a total of three years. Also, unlike 1115 waivers which require a research and evaluation component, 1915 waivers are not dependent on research.

A Growing Emphasis on Community-Based Systems

The emphasis on community-based services, demonstrated by home health in the 1960s and day health and hospice in the 1970s, has increased in the 1980s. Institutions, both skilled nursing and acute care facilities, are developing community components; and legislation at the state and federal levels consistently emphasizes community services as an alternative to institutional care. Most of the long term care demonstrations, both those described in Part II and others, including Channeling, MSSP, and S/HMO, are community-based service programs.

Medicare traditionally has not been a big reimburser of long term care, let alone community-based services. However, the 1980 Omnibus Reconciliation Act liberalized Medicare reimbursement for home health and outpatient services, allowing for the first time ongoing Medicare reimbursement for services provided by rehabilitation clinics and day centers.

The 1981 Omnibus Reconciliation Act, as noted in the previous section, moved even further to support community-based systems. In fact, Section 2176 of this act authorizes 1915 waivers, and states taking advantage of the 1915 waivers are developing or have developed programs, often legislatively-based, to offer a wide range of community-based services. A number of states also have introduced legislation to further the development of community-based services. Georgia and Minnesota, for example, have passed legislation offering, and in some cases requiring, pre-authorization screening for all institutional placements. In California, legislation recently passed proposes to give local communities control of the development of their long term care systems and calls for the integration of funding at the state level.

Relative to inpatient services, community-based services are still underdeveloped, but it is important that the pendulum not swing too far in the other direction. While in the past there has been an undue emphasis on institutional services, the institution does play an important role in long term care. There are, and probably always will be, a number of people who need institutional care and can be served best in those special facilities. Perhaps a bigger problem with the emphasis on community-based services is the implicit segregation brought about by legislation emphasizing community services. In the 1915 waivers, for example, as in many state initiatives and many of the proposed bills included in Figure 1, community-based services are emphasized and inpatient services are excluded. This segregation of the inpatient from the outpatient service system creates an artificial service environment and a potentially adversarial dichotomy. Only when the inpatient and outpatient systems become integrated into a single service system can the relative benefits of one vis-a-vis the other be fairly appraised and the most appropriate service be used.

Increasing Appreciation for the Integration of Services

The last ten or fifteen years have brought the recognition that long term care services can be addressed effectively only when both the social and medical aspects of care are encompassed. The effective nursing home and day health center already provide a mixture of social, medical and supportive services in one comprehensive package. Congregate meal, transportation, and respite care programs are increasingly being included in long term care packages, and the role of social work is becoming more accepted as a reimbursable service, both at regulatory and legislative levels.

Equally important but less developed by community-based service demonstrations has been the role of housing as another inter-related service. For the long term care population, adequate—often specially adapted—housing is as important to maintain a person in the community as are medical, social and supportive services. There has been little effort on the part of the long term care demonstrations and very little interest expressed by service funders in the reimbursement of special housing. Yet providers increasingly acknowledge that housing, either the lack or inadequacy of it in relation to need, is frequently a factor in the decision to place someone in a nursing home and in many instances has been the barrier to getting the improved aged out. Housing is a part of the institutional package and must be part of the community-based service package if programs are effectively to meet the needs of the long term care population.

The community-based long term care demonstrations all link medical, social and supportive services. In one form or another, case management is the linkage mechanism used by most of the demonstrations. In addition, some of the long term care legislation directly addresses the case coordination/case management function. For example, the 1915 waivers authorize reimbursement for those services as do a number of state initiatives, e.g., legislation in California, New York, Georgia, Minnesota and Arizona. While the importance of coordination of services is becoming increasingly recognized, different models have emerged for integrating services: case management or brokerage; and the consolidated or direct service approach.

Among the long term care demonstrations, the most popular approach for integrating services has been case management. In the case management model, it is assumed that the needed services are already available, so a case manager is added to assess needs and arrange or broker the appropriate services. As discussed in previous chapters, Triage, Project OPEN, ACCESS, the Alternative Health Services, Nursing Home Without Walls, Home Care Project and Community Long Term Care all use a variant of the brokerage model. In addition, there have been a number of more recent demonstrations which build on the concept of case management. At the state level, there are, for example, California's MSSP and Connecticut Community Care, Inc. The National Channeling demonstration also involves projects in a number of states to test a form of case management.

A second approach to the coordination of services is through a direct service or consolidated model approach. Consolidated models include service programs like health maintenance organizations, life care plans, and long term care programs like On Lok's CCODA, or for a general older population the social health maintenance organization (S/HMO) programs that are just beginning. Instead of referring to other providers, in a consolidated model the services are delivered directly by the organization consolidating services. Efforts that encourage the development of consolidated models include 1915 waivers encouraging capitation payment; California's legislation favoring a capitated, consolidated model; and the Health Care Financing Administration initiatives, including demonstrations of Average Area Per Capita Cost (AAPCC) payment for Medicare and capitation experiments in California, Minnesota and Arizona for Medicaid.

It is premature, if not inappropriate, to ask which service integration model is better. There are advantages to each and situational factors, e.g., existing service capacity in the community or level of impairment of the service population, that play important roles in determining the best model for a particular community. Moreover, these models seldom exist in pure form; most of the demonstrations deliver some services and arrange for others. The question then is not which model is better but rather what are the models' respective strengths and weaknesses and for whom and in what situation is each model most appropriate.

Broadening Entitlement for Long Term Care

One of the most critical policy issues of the 1980s and maybe years beyond is Medicare's role in long term care. Despite complaints regarding the high share of cost (coinsurance and copayment), Medicare has achieved its objective of alleviating some of the financial burden of acute care. However, with many persons now living well into old age and surviving with multiple disabilities, the ongoing high cost of long term chronic care has become the "acute" problem which today drives the older person to financial catastrophe. As noted in previous chapters, Medicaid, the guarantor of medical care to the poor, has become prime reimbursor for long term care services, and Medicare has had relatively little involvement thereby creating an anomaly: The wealthy can have whatever services money can buy, the poor are guaranteed long term care services, but the middle class must choose either to spend down their limited assets and swallow their pride in order to qualify for public health benefits or do without needed long term care assistance.

This anomaly has resulted in a basic sense of inequity to which providers and consumers are responding in counterproductive ways. For example, in some instances, the acute service system is being used to meet long term care service needs because via this mechanism providers can receive higher (Medicare) reimbursement and consumers can have lower costs. On another front, financial advisory services are now counseling their older clients to disperse their wealth before they become impaired. By so doing, formerly middle-income elderly will be eligible for public benefits yet still be able to enjoy what they have and/or preserve the family's financial resources. If Medicare were to reimburse for long term care services, especially community-based services, and reduce this financial burden further, many of these problems would be alleviated.

A number of the demonstrations have involved Medicare reimbursement. Triage, Mount Zion's Project OPEN, and On Lok's CCODA all were funded as Medicare demonstrations. In addition, in the mid-1970s Medicare experimented with reimbursement for day health and in-home services. Nevertheless, for Medicare to assume responsibility for general long term care services entails a major policy shift. As now structured, Medicare does not and cannot afford to pay for long term care services. For example, On Lok's CCODA found that in its comprehensive long term care program only 40% of its costs could be attributed to Medicare under current benefits. To expand the benefit package, Medicare as an insurance program would have to increase its revenues. More broadly put, the problem is not limited to Medicare, but reflects the need for a method of providing reimbursement for long term care services for the general older population in need of those services.

There are three ways of modifying existing health programs to cover long term care services for the general population. First, expand existing Medicare programs to include long term care services—which to some degree is already happening. A limited amount of nursing care is reimbursable under Part A benefits; some home health services are covered under Part B; and, via the 1980 Omnibus Reconciliation Act, expanded community services—both home health and professional services given through comprehensive outpatient rehabilitation facilities—are now reimbursable under Medicare. However, Medicare is, by legislative mandate, a self-supporting health insurance program; so for a significant expansion of benefits the premiums must be altered to support the increase in costs. Although some of the costs for community-based services will be offset by savings in acute medical services, wide-scale expansion of the benefit package will certainly result in increased Medicare costs and premiums.

A second approach to the funding of long term care services is through a new Medicare component. Some recently proposed legislation discusses the idea of Part D Medicare benefits which would provide reimbursement for community-based long term care services. For a separate component of Medicare, a uniquely identifiable funding base could be found, for example, a special premium or coverage through another tax base, e.g., general funds. This approach entails a new authority with additional administrative requirements and potential complications.

A third method for reducing the severe financial burden of long term care is to expand eligibility for long term care services under Medicaid. Instead of requiring immediate spend-down of almost all assets before public support is provided, a gradual spend-down of assets, as being done in a Minnesota demonstration, would reduce some of the acute financial burden on the middle-income population. Similarly, a sliding scale for long term care benefits would encourage participation of those receiving services and support their sense of self-sufficiency. While not affecting Medicare, liberalizing Medicaid eligibility can correct the inequities in the present system towards those "too rich" to qualify for Medicaid but too poor to afford the long term care services they need.

The fourth alternative is to integrate Medicare services with other long term care service funding and reimburse long term care as a single service package. This integration of long term care reimbursement is the subject of the next section.

Few people question the desirability of a comprehensive long term care system with guaranteed entitlements of all citizens to the medical, social and supportive services they require. Yet many cringe at the cost of providing such benefits, presuming that our society could never afford to provide quality long term care to all who need it. At the same time, many dollars are wasted now in providing medical services in lieu of less costly social and supportive services. The growing number of older impaired people soon will force our society to confront the demand for some long term care reimbursement for all who require it.

Integration of Funding for Long Term Care

In long term care, reimbursement has been the tail that wags the dog. Fragmented reimbursement, in large part, has been responsible for the fragmentation in services. Today many different funding sources are involved in paying for long term care services. Besides Medicaid and Medicare, Title XX and local revenues fund social services and in-home supportive services; the Older Americans Act pays for transportation, meals and some Services, and Housing and Urban Development subsidizes housing. Each of these funding programs has its own eligibility guidelines and reporting requirements—resulting in a complicated labyrinth for the impaired aged and unnecessarily high administrative costs.

Consolidation of existing reimbursement programs into a single pool of service funds would alleviate some of the access and cost problems inherent in long term care today. Consolidation of funding can be achieved at different levels—federal, state, or local project levels, and there is movement toward consolidation at all of these levels.

At the project level, most of the demonstrations described had waivers to access a single source of funds. Medicare or Medicaid and traditional billing systems were used to charge for services billable to others. One demonstration, On Lok, had Medicare waivers which authorized payment for all services regardless of the service type or the individual's entitlement. While this approach provided the single pool of funds, it was not a politically realistic solution because it put all the responsibility on Medicare, more than doubling Medicare's share of cost.

A few projects have already begun to involve multiple reimbursement sources in the funding of their demonstrations. Mount Zion tried unsuccessfully to integrate its Medicare demonstration (Project OPEN) with its state Medicaid demonstration (MSSP). Monroe County's ACCESS is bringing in some Medicare funding in a related demonstration and South Carolina's Community Long Term Care has planned Medicare involvement for discrete components of its demonstration.

The S/HMO projects, as now planned, will have Medicare and Medicaid components in their demonstrations and also include private premiums. On Lok, in its new CCODA demonstration, will have Medicare, Medicaid and private sources share the monthly capitation payment based on the individual's entitlement but without regards to service type. These attempts at funding integration are complicated, but at least for some of the demonstrations result in a single pool of funds for the delivery of all services.

At a second level, states are beginning to integrate the programs over which they have control. In California, for example, recent legislation establishes a new Department of Aging and Long Term Care integrating the many state funders of long term care into one program ultimately to be administered at the community level as a comprehensive long term care package. States, however, have no control over Medicare reimbursement. A realistic long term care reimbursement base must integrate the two large health reimbursement programs (Medicare and Medicaid) first and then add into that base private health insurance, social service benefits, special aging services, and the individual's share of cost.

At the federal level, a number of pieces of legislation are being discussed which address the integration of these different funding sources. One such mechanism is the often discussed Title XXI of the Social Security Act which consolidates all long term care service dollars from Titles XVIII, XIX and XX to establish a single long term care program. That single integrated system would be administratively simpler and more efficient due to single source accountability and streamlined eligibility. Politically, however, the system is controversial and may threaten many special interests, for it shares many characteristics with national health insurance. Some fear the universal availability of long term care services would escalate costs at a rate even higher than that seen with acute care over the last decade. Cost containment mechanisms such as risk-based capitation payment and individual share of cost can be used in said systems, however, to control costs.

The integration of funding need not occur only at the national level. For example, Medicare monies could be made available to the state for integration into a state long term care package such as proposed in California. Or funding could be integrated at the provider level.

Integration of funding, however it is accomplished, is critical to eliminating fragmentation in services, improving continuity of care, maximizing incentives for cost-effective care, and reducing the administrative cost of service delivery. On the flip side, however, it must be noted that integrating services for the long term care needy population in essence creates another funding source—one which separates the impaired from the rest of the population. Ultimately, true integration would involve a single service system for all people, guaranteeing all individuals the services they need with consumer and provider incentives for effective and efficient use.

Use of Risk-Based Capitation Reimbursement

The traditional health care system in the United States has been criticized for its lack of cost controls. According to that system, a recipient, as the first party, receives services from a provider, the second party, with all costs paid by an insurer, the third party. In this system, neither the recipient nor the service provider has an incentive for cost control. As an alternative to this model, a new model of health care reimbursement has begun to emerge involving capitation payments with provider assumption of financial risk. According to this model, the individual or the funding agency pays the provider a fixed amount or premium for which the provider agrees to deliver all needed health services.

There are three service models now operating—or proposed—using risk-based capitation: the HMO, S/HMO, and the CCODA. In the medical field the health maintenance organization—the HMO—is the best known. The HMO is built upon the premise that a small fee from a large number of healthy people can be used to cover the total cost of health care for the few who need it. The HMO provides primarily medical services, but there is an incentive to provide education and preventive services to reduce higher cost medical care. With the provider responsible for the cost of services, it is argued that there is a built-in incentive to control health care costs. Generally HMOs have been able to provide better control over the cost of health care delivery as compared to traditional health insurance programs. In essence, this is a form of health insurance, in which the provider of services is assuming financial responsibility for service delivery.

In focusing on a generally healthy population, HMOs have usually avoided the aged fearing their greater needs and higher risks. But innovative HMOs and others are starting new programs applying the principles of the HMO to the field of aging and long term care. The Medicare capitation demonstrations in the early 1980s have shown that Medicare capitation payments below Medicare costs (Average Area Per Capita Cost or AAPCC) combined with the HMO premium can allow an HMO to expand Medicare and eliminate the individual's coinsurance and copayment responsibilities for Medicare

A and B services (Greenlick, Lamb, Carpenter, Fischer, Marks, & Cooper, 1983). Provisions of the 1982 Tax Equity and Fiscal Responsibility Act will extend this program to other interested HMO's.

The S/HMO, or social health maintenance organization, builds upon the concept of the HMO, but focuses the model on an older population, 65+ years of age. Like the HMO, the S/HMO receives a single premium as payment in full for all health services. Unlike the HMO, the S/HMO explicitly includes in its package social and supportive services often required by the older population. The S/HMO, like the HMO, is predicated on the fact that most of the participants will be healthy and the savings in service costs to the healthy will offset the cost of long term care for the impaired. As now planned, however, the S/HMO sites will receive a higher Medicare rate for the frail (frailty adjusted AAPCC) and also offer an expanded long term care package through Medicaid; they also will be allowed to exclude long term care costs above a predetermined level.

The CCODA uses the principle of risk-based capitation but focuses on a still narrower and smaller population of institutionally certified frail aged. It applies the management and financing principles of the HMO to a high cost population. The monthly premium is higher, reflecting the greater service need of the population, and the provider is responsible for meeting all health and social service needs of that population in return for that premium. The monthly premium is the same for all individuals. Medicare, Medicaid and the individual all share the cost of the premium based on the individual's entitlement. While the CCODA does not have the opportunity to benefit from premium payments from a large number of healthy people, it does have, by focusing on an already expensive population, a greater opportunity for cost savings. By substituting community services for high cost inpatient services and eliminating the administrative costs of fee-for-service billing to multiple reimbursers, cost savings can be maximized.

All three of these risk-based capitation models have put the provider at risk for the control of costs. Capitation payment does provide an opportunity for integrating multiple funding sources, can reduce administrative requirements and paperwork of service delivery, and can give the provider freedom and flexibility over the use of alternative, cost-effective services. On a minus side, however, capitation programs do restrict the individual's freedom of choice, forcing the service recipient to go to one organization for all health and health-related services. It has also been argued that the consolidated approach gives the provider too much control over services since the provider is paid whether or not any services are delivered. With the greater freedom over services afforded in the consolidated model goes a commensurate increase in provider responsibility. The unethical provider can neglect the impaired aged and let them die. Quality control procedures and outside review as required of any service provider, as well as the individual consumer's right to disenroll or file a grievance, are necessary protection to ensure that the level of care provided, meets or exceeds existing standards. As long as the responsible provider has no "out," that is, cannot discharge an individual who becomes too frail (and expensive), the provider will have an incentive to provide social and supportive services to offset the higher costs of acute and institutional care.

There is great interest on the part of policy makers and reimbursement agencies towards fixed cost, risk-based reimbursement as a cost control measure. Such a system can be abused if funding agencies set the rates unrealistically low or irresponsible providers take advantage of the system. However, the biggest impediment to risk-based reimbursement for long term care is the reluctance of existing providers to assume financial risk. Responsible long term care providers who want the freedom and flexibility to deliver services in response to individual needs rather than reimbursement agency constraints must realize that it is the provider assumption of financial risk which is the cost of freedom.

Competitive Models of Care

Essentially, there are two schools of thought regarding the role of competition in health care delivery. Some believe that a single service protected from competition can become inefficient, ineffectual and ultimately unresponsive to the needs of those being served; instead, health service delivery should be treated like any other industry with multiple providers encouraged to compete for the health dollar to get the best value. Others argue that competition can be expensive and destructive and that the cost of marketing and the game playing involved, e.g., bait and switch, can become abusive to the individual consumer; and since setting up a health delivery system is so expensive, our society cannot afford to have multiple competitors, each with their own expensive facilities and equipment such as CAT scanners. Instead, health care should be a regulated industry like a utility, with a single health system designed in response to the needs of the community. There are merits to both arguments and perhaps a balance between the two approaches is most effective.

The role of competition is in part dependent on the nature of the program: a service provider is more likely to face competition than is a statewide nursing home pre-authorization screening project. However, community-based long term care is a new frontier and it is important that in these early stages new demonstrations be open and willing to share their methods and their experiences. In most cases, demonstration projects are already competing with the existing service system; strong competition from other demonstrations would be destructive in these early stages when the programs are just developing. However, innovation is the lifeblood of a dynamic system, and no service environment or community should ever prohibit the development of new solutions.

Individual and Family Responsibility

Much of the discussion in this report has focused on public funding sources for long term care. Yet individuals and their families and friends today assume a large share of the responsibility for the cost and services required by the older population. Again, there are different views: some argue that society should take responsibility for all essential services to its population, while others feel that the individual and/or his or her family must assume responsibility for their own needs. In this debate, there are two distinct issues—the individual's cost responsibility for long term care and the role of family in the care of the older person.

No one questions or wishes to undermine the individual's assumed financial responsibility for meeting his or her own needs. Safety and security needs are basically provided by society. For meeting less predictable high cost medical needs, there are public (Medicare) and private insurance programs. However, if an individual lacks resources, our society implicitly guarantees—through Medicaid, public health programs and county hospitals—essential medical services. For other basic needs, like housing and food, the individual is presumed responsible although some public assistance programs are available, e.g., HUD housing subsidies, food stamps and congregate meal programs.

Long term care involves the blending of many needs—medical, social, supportive, and housing—blurring the issue of entitlements and societal support guarantees. The current operating premise is that the individual has full financial responsibility for long term care services until personal resources are exhausted, at which time public programs assume the uncovered cost. This system creates inequities and disincentives. A long term care needy person living in the community typically has the responsibility to find special housing and meet unusual nutritional needs. There is no reimbursement for those services because they are not medical. If that same person were in a nursing home, all of these services could be included as part of the medical long term care package. Medical insurance programs are concerned about these broader multiple needs of the long term care client and severely limit long term care benefits. Medical services "safety net" programs, e.g., Medicaid, could not escape long term care and have found themselves paying for medical, social and supportive services.

Financial participation in a service program increases the individual's sense of responsibility and is desirable. Medicare programs involve coinsurance and copayment for some share of the covered services. Even HMOs require some token payment for certain services as a disincentive to unnecessarily high utilization. The task is to structure financial participation in such a way that it does not break the person or deter access to medical service. One approach would be to distinguish health care-related costs (medical services and health-related supportive services such as personal care and special diets) from normal living expenses (room and board). Existing health reimbursement programs could be expanded to cover the health care costs in inpatient or community settings with financial participation covered through health insurance premiums and/or modest copayments for services. Normal living expenses, even the board and care costs of the skilled nursing facility, would remain an individual responsibility with social service and income programs providing the safety net.

The role of family involvement for care of the older person also presents difficult problems. No one would want to replace the services provided by family and friends with a formal network of services. However, the notion that family and friends can replace the long term care system simply is not realistic. Not everyone has the family and friends to give that little bit of help needed to live in the community. In addition, family and friends, when present, have many other responsibilities; additional responsibilities for the care of the older parent often prove to be the last straw, breaking down family networks and disenfranchising parents and their children. In some cases, the family member may be a slightly less frail spouse; the added demand for care of the partner often results in health services for two, rather than one. In the present health system, family members are often forced either to accept the heavy burden of care or abandon their relatives who need long term care and deal with the guilt. If there could be some assistance and support to alleviate acute demands so they can provide continuing support on a longer basis, families would not be forced to send their frail relatives to a total care facility. A realistic balance is needed to build upon the natural support networks of family and friends and provide formal services that support and complement these networks, helping the older impaired person lead as full and independent a life as possible.

In this political environment, the pendulum has turned toward greater emphasis on individual and family responsibility for long term care services. These last few paragraphs have just scratched the surface of this important area, and much more will be said in the years ahead. It is not a simple matter of deciding individual versus societal responsibility but rather the need for rational, effective and equitable systems for balancing the needs of the individual, the family, the community and society as a whole.

CONCLUSION

In the field of long term care, there are problems and questions but few answers. Perhaps a useful way of looking at the issues and movements in long term care is to think of the different arguments as being end points of a scale, with a workable solution somewhere between the extremes. The end points related to long term care include institutional versus community services, centralized systems of reimbursement versus very localized control over resources, consolidated versus brokerage models of service, full societal responsibility for all human services versus individual responsibility.

The demonstrations described in this monograph were initiated to correct some perceived imbalance in the existing system. Although today the problems of long term care are larger because of the change in demographics, many solutions that are being discussed and practiced are not new. Case management as a concept was first discussed in 1902. Community care was a norm in the early 1900s when the inpatient facility and later the nursing home became the innovative alternative. However, once systems become the norm, become bureaucratized and lose the ability to change, they become ineffectual. What is needed is a mechanism that encourages change and innovation, a means that allows programs to seek new solutions continually.

Today, the momentum is towards increased community control and provider assumption of risk, with a constant concern for cost containment. While these directions and goals may change over time, programs can be given a structure that fosters appropriate organizational change and renewal. The concept of the community laboratory—discussed in Chapter 11—offers such a structure. The community laboratory could be an ongoing tool whereby communities are given responsibility and control over their resources, are monitored in terms of the quality of services they provide, and are trained to use information to continue to change and develop. In turn, the community laboratory approach may result in a dynamic environment where long term care services are not so much a defined system, but a dynamic, ever-changing model of service delivery.

REFERENCE

Greenlick, M. R., Lamb, S. J., Carpenter, T. M., Jr., Fischer, T. S., Marks, S. D., & Cooper, W. J. Kaiser-Permanente's Medicare Plus Project: A successful Medicare prospective payment demonstration. *Health Care Financing Reviw,* 1983, *4,* 85-97.